Building Health

Immune system disorders are rampant in our society—running the gamut from frequent respiratory infections to AIDS and breast cancer. This invaluable herbal handbook concentrates on the more common everyday ailments including candidiasis, chronic fatigue, herpes simplex, urinary tract infections and ever-returning colds and flus.

Writing from the premise that human immunity is an interface between individuals and their environment, the author, a gifted herbalist, shows how the foundation of good health is a healthy lifestyle and describes the crucial role herbal medicine can play in immune system health by supporting every organ and cell in the body.

D1569867

About the Author

Gail Ulrich is founder and director of Blazing Star Herbal School in Shelburne Falls, Massachusetts and owner of New England Botanicals herbal products. An herbalist for more than 20 years and a certified Flower Essence Practitioner and Instructor, Gail has organized the Annual Women's Herbal Conference in New England for the past 10 years, and is an organizer of the Healing With Flowers Conference as well as many other herbal events. She teaches nationally, and has helped formulate several lines of herbal products. She brings her love of the herbal world, wealth of personal experience and passion for teaching to all her work.

MEDICINE
THE 21 CENTURY

HERBS TO BOOST IMMUNITY

*Herbal tonics to keep you healthy
and strong including echinacea,
Siberian ginseng, astragalus and more*

Gail Ulrich

Keats Publishing, Inc. ✦ New Canaan, Connecticut

HERBS TO BOOST IMMUNITY

Copyright © 1997 by Gail Ulrich

Library of Congress Cataloging-in-Publication Data

Ulrich, Gail.
  Herbs to boost immunity / Gail Ulrich.
    p.   cm.
  Includes bibliographical references and index.
  ISBN 0-87983-864-7
  1. Herbs—Therapeutic use.   2. Immunity—Popular works.   I.
Title.
RM666.H3U44   1997
615'.321—dc21   97-27730
                                                               CIP

Printed in the United States of America

Good Herb Guides are published by
Keats Publishing, Inc.
27 Pine Street (Box 876)
New Canaan, Connecticut 06840-0876

98 97 96   6 5 4 3 2 1

Contents

To my dad, Dr. Sanford S. Ulrich, D.C. whose pioneering vision of natural healing illumined my path.

Acknowledgements
Thanks to Don Cerow, Lilian Jackman, Linda Patterson and Saretta Ulrich for their help with this book.

Introduction

"Man did not weave the web of life. He is but a strand in it. Whatever befalls the Earth, befalls the sons [and daughters] of the Earth."—**Chief Seattle**

Although each individual comes into this life with certain genetic strengths and weaknesses, we all have the ability to be truly well. Yet more and more 20th-century Americans are succumbing to immune system ailments— from colds and flu, herpes and chronic fatigue to AIDS and breast cancer.

At the same time, the pollution of the Earth has reached an alarming level. With the Industrial Revolution and the mass production which followed, devitalized packaged foods began replacing fresh natural foods; thousands of chemicals, many of them toxic, have permeated our food, air and water. The rapid increase in immune disorders clearly coincides with the increase in environmental disorders.

At the same time that we attend to our personal health, we must begin the enormous task of cleaning up our polluted environment. If it is true that we are microcosms of this macrocosm, the Earth, then we can start on a personal level by buying organically grown foods, using biodegradable products for household chores and recycling. And as we clean up our environment, it is clear that we will in effect be rebuilding our own immune systems.

From this perspective, it becomes clear that human immunity is an interface between individuals and their environment. And while lifestyle changes and a healthy diet are the underlying essentials for immune system health, herbal medicine can play a complementary role in enhancing immunity by supporting every organ and cell in the body.

THE MIND-BODY CONNECTION

On a biological level, immunity is a complex process that happens within the body, involving many organ systems and physiological processes rather than one specific group of organs. Recent research has shown that immunity is much more than a physiological process and that immune cells are in both the cardiovascular and digestive systems. We know too, that immune function is negatively influenced by stress, low self-esteem, poor diet, lack of exercise, smoking, drinking and drugs and is positively influenced by a healthy lifestyle, an optimistic outlook and affirmations.

For nearly 20 years, the science of psychoneuroimmunology (body-mind-immune system interactions) has shown us that every thought we have influences the immune system. A vast amount of information has come out showing the connection between the mind and healing. It is now clear that depression, which has reached almost epidemic proportions, directly affects a person's ability to heal and weakens the immune system as well. According to Dr. C. Norman Shealy, more illnesses involve the immune system than all other body systems combined. Studies at Harvard Medical School show us that illness is four times more likely to occur after a stressful experience.

The notion that the mind and emotions can more powerfully influence the body than physical stressors is illustrated in the following study. Two groups were followed, the first was made up of heavy smokers who felt loved in their relationships; the second was nonsmokers who felt very lonely and depressed. Surprisingly, the happy smokers had a significantly lower incidence of illness than the unhappy nonsmokers. The more we live in the present moment, the better our relationships, and the more faith we have in our own ability to heal, the more effective herbs, flower essences, homeopathy and other forms of natural healing will be and the stronger our immune system will become.

Super Foods:
The Immune Diet

The typical American diet is overloaded with processed foods: cold cereal or a bagel for breakfast, a burger or ham sandwich on white bread with chips or fries plus coffee or a soda for lunch, and meat and potatoes, pizza or pasta and maybe a salad of iceberg lettuce for dinner. This all adds up to a devitalized diet high in simple carbohydrates, saturated fats and lots of calories and low in nutrient-rich vegetables, fruits and whole grains. It's no wonder that Americans are generally overweight and undernourished.

An immune-enhancing diet would include a wide variety of colorful, real foods as close to their natural state as possible: organically grown fruits and vegetables, whole grains and legumes along with adequate amounts of protein from soy, fish or grains.

Commercially raised meat and poultry are commonly treated with drugs and hormones. These contaminants create toxicity in the body, weakening immunity and are often cofactors in many illnesses from allergies to hormonal imbalance. It is far healthier for the immune system to minimize your consumption of animal products and to restrict your consumption to that which is naturally raised.

Certain nutrient-dense foods, especially organic vegetables, fruits and whole grains, show a remarkable ability to increase vitality and enhance immunity. Also, natural yogurt with live cultures can help to repopulate the intestine with a garden of beneficial intestinal flora, restoring digestive health. Taking *Lactobacillus acidophilus* in yogurt or tablet form has been shown to increase general immunity, help heal infections and restore metabolic health. Yogurt made from goat's milk is much more easily digested than that made from cow's milk.

Not enough can be said about the value of garlic and onions in a healing diet for the immune system. Besides their cholesterol-lowering and antibiotic effects and their blood pressure-regulating and cardiovascular benefits, these allium family foods help to detoxify the body from chemicals and drugs. For example, a good preventive dose of garlic would be three crushed, fresh cloves daily. Bear in mind though, that because of its blood-thinning capabilities, it is not advisable to take garlic when there is risk of hemorrhage.

Miso soup, the classic favorite of macrobiotic cooks, is a fine food for speeding recovery from illness and restoring strength and vitality. Made from fermented soy bean paste, it is easily digested and is delicious with onions, carrots and dark leafy greens.

Another powerful restorative soup highly acclaimed in both Jewish and Chinese traditions is chicken soup. Many versions are available: one of them is given in this book. Usually, the bones (which include the marrow) are cooked in the soup along with a panoply of tonic herbs and vegetables. Tofu is an easily digested protein which can also be used in soup recipes or added to other dishes.

Both medicinal mushrooms and sea vegetables have a place of high honor in the Oriental tradition and are being used more commonly now in Western culture as well for their numerous healing benefits for the immune system. Shiitake and maitake are two delicious mushrooms which are often available in the produce section of supermarkets. Both of these can be prepared by cooking them with onions, garlic and other vegetables or adding them to soups and stews.

Some delicious recipes for enchancing immunity follow.

Garlic-Ginger Sesame Sauce

A wonderfully spicy sauce to use on cooked vegetables, grains, pasta or entrees, it is useful for decongesting colds and easing scratchy throats.

    10 to 13 cloves organic garlic
    ½ cup sesame butter or tahini
    1-inch piece ginger root, grated
    4 teaspoons dark toasted sesame oil
    ¼ cup tamari or shoyu soy sauce
    Juice of 1 organic lemon and grated peel
    Honey (to taste)

Blend all ingredients in a food processor or blender. As sauce will be thick, dilute it with water to gravy consistency. Add a little honey to mellow flavors.

When my parents were seeking a tasty alternative to salt for seasoning their food, I created the following recipe.

Super Immune Tune Seasoning

    2 parts kelp powder
    1 part nettle seeds
    2 parts toasted sesame seeds
    ¼ part nettle leaf
    2 parts milk thistle seeds
    1 part thyme
    ½ part garlic granules
    ½ part oregano
    ½ part marjoram
    2 parts basil
    1 pinch cayenne powder (optional)
    1 part alfalfa

Grind the sesame seeds and milk thistle seeds in a spice mill or coffee grinder. Add the rest of the ingredients and mix well. Put into a spice shaker and use liberally, as a super-food supplement on cooked vegetable dishes, salads, grains and pasta dishes.

Shot-gun Smoothie

2 cups organic tomato or vegetable juice
1-2 cloves garlic
1 teaspoon horseradish, fresh-grated (or ½ teaspoon powder)
1 gram powdered vitamin C
50,000 units vitamin A (from beta carotene)
A dash of ground ginger
A dash of Worcestershire sauce
A dash of cayenne powder
A little lemon juice and honey

Blend all ingredients in a blender. This tastes like a very spicy Bloody Mary (without the alcohol) and is great for relieving cold symptoms and winter maladies.

Thanks to my dear friend, Rosemary Gladstar for the following recipe. This wonderfully warming drink has relieved many a head cold and soothed many sore throats.

Hot Ginger Lemonade

1 cup fresh ginger root,   1 fresh lemon, squeezed
   chopped   Honey to taste
1 quart water

Place ginger root in a nonmetal pot. Cover with the water. Simmer 10 to 15 minutes. Remove from heat and add fresh-squeezed lemons and honey to taste. Sprinkle with a few grains of cayenne for an extra spicy zest.

The following tonic soup recipe is rather like a bouillon. It is beneficial as part of a holistic treatment for deep immune disorders.

Fu Zheng Tang Bouillon

6 astragalus root slices
8 to 10 codonopsis root slices
1 handful atractylodes rhizome pieces
2–4 ounces reishi mushroom chopped
1–2 ounces Siberian ginseng pieces
1 handful shiitake mushrooms
Organic turkey bones (or miso)
1–2 cups each, organic carrots and celery

Cook all dried herbs, mushrooms and turkey bones in 10 cups of water for 72 hours on a slow simmer. (If you are vegetarian, omit turkey bones and add miso to taste after the soup is fully cooked.) In the last hour of cooking, add carrots and celery. Let soup cool. Strain, and freeze in ice-cube trays. One serving is one cube, melted, once a day. The first four ingredients can be obtained through Herbalist and Alchemist. See Herbal Suppliers, page 86.

Three Ways to
Build Immunity

According to most clinically trained herbalists, there are three ways to build immunity. These three protocols help to fine-tune herbal therapy to the needs of the individual.

1. Simple immune imbalances such as colds, flu, mild infections and those conditions that are not deep-seated, but come and go fairly quickly, are treated with surface immune herbs or secretory herbs, such as echinacea, garlic, pau d'arco and milk thistle. These herbs increase the protective ability of the mucous membranes and stimulate the production of white blood cells. By working with the macrophages, these plants strengthen the secretory immune system. When there is lowered resistance rather than long-term immune depression, this class of herbs works quickly and effectively.

2. When there is long-term stress on the immune system and its deeper reserves become depleted, many people develop immune deficiency. This is usually caused by a combination of many factors operating over a long period of time rather than one specific thing; it does not happen suddenly or overnight. For example, an individual who must perform at maximum potential during the day but gets less than an adequate amount of sleep, eats a nutrient-depleted fast-food diet, suffers from indigestion and is not happy at work is a prime candidate for deep immune deficiency.

Although there may be no specific physical complaint,

the underlying immune system is affected and the person may lack energy and *joie de vivre*. In this case, deep immune-system tonic herbs or those herbs that build the bone marrow reserve would be used. Nourishing foods or superfoods such as garlic, blue-green algae and sea vegetables would be good choices. Some of the herbs that fall into the category of deep immune system tonics are astragalus, shiitake mushrooms, Siberian ginseng and milk thistle.

Because herbs have a multitude of constituents, it is not uncommon for an herb such as milk thistle or echinacea to be useful as both a surface immune-system herb as well as a deep immune-system tonic or even as an adaptogen, which brings us to the third category of immune system herbs.

3. The third way to build immunity focuses on herbs classified as adaptogens. An adaptogen strengthens and normalizes the hormonal function of the body. This term was coined by the renowned Russian scientist, I. I. Brekhman, who researched Siberian ginseng (*Eleutherococcus senticosus*) extensively for 30 years and developed the three criteria for adaptogens described below.

First, an adaptogenic herb must cause no harm and put no additional stress on the body. The second criterion is that the herb should help the body to cope with a wide variety of environmental, physical and psychological stresses. And thirdly, it must have a nonspecific action on the body. This means that it must address many issues rather than a specific symptom. An adaptogen works by helping the body to conserve energy and to cope with stress. Some common adaptogens are Siberian ginseng, Panax ginseng, reishi mushroom, milk thistle and licorice. An individual experiencing high levels of stress because of a new job, a divorce, or moving will have lowered resistance and be more susceptible to illness. In these situations, adaptogenic herbs are of great benefit.

Recent immune system study shows that the nervous

system and hormonal system are linked to the immune system and that these three systems strongly affect each other. It's no wonder then, that many women experience mood swings and lowered resistance around their menstrual cycle. Clearly, stress creates many changes in the hormonal system. High stress levels cause an increase in the production of the hormones cortisol and adrenaline, both of which lower immune function. Adaptogenic herbs help the body to cope with a wide variety of biological and environmental stresses.

Exercise

It has been said that exercise can do even more for a person's health and well-being than diet. In addition to keeping the body flexible, slowing the aging process, improving digestion and circulation, reducing stress, depression, fatigue and body weight, exercise improves immunity and brings with it a sense of vitality. In addition, sweating can help cleanse the body by eliminating wastes. It is always important to increase one's level of activity gradually, and to practice deep breathing while exercising. A brisk 20- to 30-minute walk at least three times a week is enough to make a significant difference.

Regular exercise also helps the body to speed recovery from many ailments including some types of arthritis, digestive and stress-related illnesses. Choosing an enjoyable exercise is essential. For example, if you don't like lifting weights or running on a treadmill at the gym, choose swing dancing, volleyball or yoga—whatever brings you joy.

For those who are bedridden because of an immune system ailment, gentle yoga postures and yogic breathing can be done lying down and can prevent loss of vitality, constipation and muscle atrophy. These postures should be done slowly and carefully, depending upon level of strength and wellness. Those who feel any pain or cramping should stop and proceed more gently next time.

Making Your Own
Herbal Preparations

Besides the deep satisfaction that comes from making your own herbal preparations, it is more cost-effective. Someone with a chronic immune condition can easily use up a one-ounce bottle of tincture in a matter of days. Assuming that you will need to take your herbal formula for a minimum of three weeks, and sometimes up to six months or a year, at $7 to $12 per ounce, this can quickly become quite expensive. Furthermore, when you make your own herbal preparations, you are participating in your own healing process. There are many ways to prepare herbal remedies. The ones given here are simple and effective.

Teas

There are two methods of preparing teas: infusions and decoctions. Infusions are made by steeping: decoctions are simmered.

Infusions: Make infusions of the delicate parts of plants, such as flowers and leaves. A simple infusion can be made by using 1 to 2 teaspoons of dried herbs for each cup of tea you intend to make. Place the herbs into a nonmetal teapot or canning jar with a lid. Pour in 1 cup of boiling water for each cup of tea. Place the lid on the pot and steep for 10 to 20 minutes. Strain and drink. An infusion can be taken hot or cold and sweetened with honey, maple syrup, natural sugar (like Sucanat) or with sweet herbs such as licorice or stevia.

A strong infusion is made by placing 1 ounce of dried flowers or leaves into a 1-quart canning jar (which is made of tempered glass and can withstand boiling water) or other nonmetal container. Pour just-boiled water in to fill the jar and fasten the lid tightly. This prevents the volatile constituents from escaping. Steep for 15 to 30 minutes. Some herbs can be steeped longer, depending upon the plant constituents. Strain and compost the spent herbs. Drink ½ to 1 cup of tea two to three times a day. If you don't drink all the tea right away, store any extra in the refrigerator for up to three days.

An ingenious way to make an infusion is in a French press coffee maker (available in most department stores and specialty coffee shops). Place the herbs in the French press pot and pour boiling water over them to fill the coffee maker. After 15 to 30 minutes, press the plunger down, pushing the herbs to the bottom of the pot. Pour out the infusion as you would coffee. You can pour the infusion into a thermos bottle so you can have warm tea to drink throughout the day. An automatic tea-maker is also now available. Produced by the same company that makes Mr. Coffee coffee makers, this one is aptly called Mrs. Tea.

Decoctions: Decoctions are usually made from the tougher, denser parts of plants, such as roots, barks, seeds and berries. The standard method for making a decoction is to put one ounce of dried herbs into a nonmetal pot (enamel, tempered glass, Pyrex or Corningware). Pour one quart of cold water over the herbs and cover with a well-fitting lid. Bring to a simmer over very low heat, and simmer for 15 to 30 minutes. Strain out the herbs and compost them. Drink ½ to 1 cup of decoction two to three times a day.

An alternate method is to start with a strong infusion of herbs, which has been strained. Place the strained infusion into a pot and simmer on the lowest possible heat until the liquid is reduced by half. (If you started with 2 cups of infusion, you now have 1 cup of decoction.) To make a double decoction, start with a decoction and simmer it on the lowest possible heat until the decoction is reduced by half. Strain and drink. This double decoction will be much stronger and more concentrated than the original decoction, so smaller doses will be effective. A double decoction is a good base from which to make a syrup. If you are new to the world of herbs, try each method for making decoctions and decide which one works best for you.

If you have an automatic drip coffee maker, you can also streamline the decoction-making process. Place the herbs in the bottom of the coffee maker instead of on top, where the coffee usually goes. Add water to the top of the machine and let the preheated water run down over the herbs. Let the decoction sit on the warmer for 20 to 30 minutes and then strain. You can pour this decoction into a thermos, and take it to work with you or keep it in a covered jar in the refrigerator for up to three days.

TINCTURES

Also called extracts, tinctures are concentrated herbal preparations which usually use alcohol as a solvent and sometimes glycerin or vinegar. A tincture is an effective way to take a remedy. Tinctures are quick-acting and dissolve almost all of the plant constituents, since alcohol-based tinctures are a mixture of both alcohol and water. Although alcohol-based tinctures are the most effective, glycerin and sometimes vinegar tinctures are appropriate for those who are unable to use alcohol-based preparations. Furthermore, tinctures are often a more convenient way to take herbs than brewing up a pot of tea. Making your own tinctures is easy, cost-effective and a good way to preserve fresh herbs for an indefinite period of time, since most tinctures can last decades without losing quality.

Alcohol-Based Tinctures: To make a tincture from dried herbs, use the woody or dense parts of herbs for the best tinctures. Place 1 part dried herbs in a blender or food processor, and shred or chop into small pieces (but don't powder them). Put the chopped herbs into an 8-ounce glass jar with a tight-fitting lid. Pour 5 parts 40- to 50-percent alcohol (80 to 100 proof) over the herbs. The liquid used in the tincture is called the *menstruum*. Vodka or brandy work well. If you can purchase grain alcohol (190 proof: 95 percent alcohol) in your state, dilute it with 50 percent water. For example, if using grain alcohol, pour 2-½ cups of alcohol into a quart jar and fill to the top with water.

Shake the container every day for at least two weeks to evenly mix the herbs and alcohol. If the herbs absorb some of the solvent, add a little more. After two to six weeks, strain the herbal tincture through a large piece of cheesecloth or muslin and squeeze out as much liquid as possible. I like to use canning jars so I can place the cloth over the jar and screw the metal ring over the cloth to make straining easier. A tincture press works best; see Appendix for places to purchase a press. Compost the spent herbs, known as *marc*. Store your finished tincture in a dark glass bottle with a lid or stopper. Label with the name of the herb, part used, date and strength of alcohol. Store in a cool place away from direct light. Refrigeration is not necessary.

When tincturing fragile parts of plants, such as leaves

and flowers, fresh herbs generally make a better preparation, but roots and dense plant parts can be used fresh, too. Place fresh herbs in a blender or food processor, or chop finely. Fill a jar with fresh, chopped herbs, leaving about an inch of room at the top of the jar. Pour alcohol over the herbs (as described above), filling the jar to the top so that the alcohol completely covers the herbs. Follow the rest of the instructions given for tincturing dried herbs.

Glycerin-Based Tinctures: Glycerin-based tinctures are sweet-tasting and milder than alcohol tinctures, making them a good choice for children and those who cannot tolerate alcohol. They are less potent than alcohol tinctures, though, and don't extract resinous or oily herbs very well. Vegetable glycerin is a sweet, mucilaginous liquid, derived from plant sources. Purchase vegetable glycerin from your natural food store or through some of the resources listed at the back of this book. Glycerites are best stored in the refrigerator and last up to two years.

To make a tincture with glycerin (called a "glycerite"), using dried herbs, grind 4 ounces of herbs in your blender or food processor. Put herbs in a 16-ounce jar. Mix together: 1-½ cups of vegetable glycerin and ½ cup of distilled water. Pour this mixture over the herbs. Secure the lid tightly and shake the jar daily. Follow the directions listed above for tincturing. If you want to make a glycerite from fresh herbs, follow the same guidelines for tincturing fresh herbs, as described above, but instead of alcohol, use a mixture of 75 percent glycerin and 25 percent water.

Herbal Vinegars: Vinegar-based tinctures are the least desirable. Vinegar is not a very good solvent and has a short shelf life (about a year), depending upon the acetic acid of the vinegar. I prefer to make herbal vinegars with culinary herbs, such as rosemary, thyme, basil or garlic, or mineral-rich herbs like dandelion, nettles or raspberry leaf. Herbal vinegars are best made from apple cider vinegar and used on salads or for other culinary use.

Fill a glass jar with fresh herbs and cover with vinegar. Secure tightly with a nonmetal lid or stopper (vinegar corrodes metal). Place in direct sunlight or in a warm place for two to six weeks. Strain. Store in a cupboard away from light in a glass jar with a nonmetal lid.

CAPSULES

Herb capsules can be purchased in a natural food store or you can make your own to insure good quality. Keep herbs as whole as possible to preserve their volatile principles and medicinal properties. When ready to use, grind herbs in a coffee or spice grinder until they are powdered. Wear a pollen mask to avoid exposure to herb dust, which can irritate lungs and nasal passages. Two-part gelatin capsules, as well as vegetarian capsules are available in three sizes from a natural food store or mail-order source, listed in the Appendix. Capsule sizes range from "0" (largest) to "00" and "000" (smallest). An "00" capsule holds about 600 mg. Open the empty capsule and scoop the herb powder into it. Close the capsule. Mechanical capping devices are available in some natural food stores or through many herb companies by mail-order. These devices hold multiple capsules in place for faster filling.

INFUSED OILS

Many herbs can be extracted in oil and applied topically for skin ailments like eczema or psoriasis, for wound-healing, a chest rub or ear infection. For medicinal purposes, olive oil is the best solvent.

To make an infused herbal oil, place 8 ounces of dried herbs in a clean, dry pint jar. Add olive oil to one inch above the level of the herbs in the jar. Cover with a well-fitting lid, but don't tighten it completely. Place the jar in a warm place (on top of a refrigerator or water heater) for two to four weeks or place in a saucepan of water on low heat for three days, or in the sun for ten days. The ideal temperature during infusion is 75 to 100 degrees F. After the appropriate length of time, strain the oil through cheesecloth and compost the marc (spent herbs). Store the herbal oil in a jar with a tight-fitting lid in a cool, dark place. Label it as described in the directions for making tinctures. You can also add a few drops of essential oil, such as chamomile, lemon, tea tree or a combination of patchouli and sandalwood to the infused oil to help preserve it. It will keep about a year.

Fresh herbs can also be used to make infused oils, but they tend to mold because of the water content. If you are using fresh herbs, wilt them overnight first to eliminate some of the water and then chop them finely. Pack the jar with fresh herbs, leaving an inch of headroom at the top. Add olive oil, to one inch above the level of the herbs. Use a wooden chopstick or a knife to poke down into the jar, releasing any air, so that the herbs are completely submerged and surrounded by oil. This helps to insure that the oil will not spoil. Follow the rest of the directions above.

When straining the oil, don't wring or squeeze the herbs, as this will introduce water into the oil. After straining, let the oil sit undisturbed for a day. Since oil floats on water, the water will settle to the bottom of the jar. Carefully siphon off the water with a turkey baster and discard it. Removing this water will prevent the oil from fermenting. Add a few drops of essential oil, vitamin E or propolis extract to preserve it further.

SALVES

A convenient way to apply herbs topically is with a salve. Salves can be used for healing cracked dry skin, rashes, abrasions and more. Don't use salves on fungal skin conditions, since fungus, like yeast, thrives in a warm, moist environment, and salves hold warmth and moisture in the skin.

Start with an infused herbal oil. Place 8 ounces of herbal oil in a clean, dry nonmetal pan. Add ¼ cup of beeswax. Heat together over very low heat, stirring occasionally, until the beeswax is completely melted. Test the consistency by placing a few drops of this mixture on a cold china plate. Check the firmness of your salve. If it is too soft, add a little more beeswax; if too hard, add more oil. When it has reached the right consistency, pour the salve into small glass containers or tins and cool until firm. When stored in a cool, dark place, salves will last for many months, even years.

Materia Medica for the Immune System

The world of herbs offers a multitude of green allies for enhancing immunity. In every culture around the globe, herbs have been used for thousands of years as the primary form of health care. Unlike drugs, herbs address more than just the biochemical aspects of immunity. From teas and tinctures to foods and flower essences, herbs embody the energy and spirit of a plant and correspond to human energetic patterns.

A concise listing of herbs to enhance immunity would be nearly impossible, since a great many aspects of immunity are addressed by literally hundreds of herbs. The herbs listed here represent those that cover a broad spectrum of immune ailments and are fairly easy to obtain.

Astragalus *(Astragalus membranaceus)*
Part used: Root
Actions: Antitumor, energy tonic, stops sweating
Indications: Although there are about 200 species of astragalus that are native to the United States, most are toxic and it is only *Astragalus membranaceus* that is used medicinally. A Chinese species of milk vetch (a pea family plant), astragalus has been used for thousands of years in the Orient. Frequently used as an immune system stimulant and as a general tonic herb for the common cold, astragalus is used as a deep immune system tonic, much like echinacea.

Like echinacea, it increases the proliferation and activity

of immuno-competent cells. In Traditional Chinese Medicine (TCM), it is often simmered in chicken soup along with other herbs to make a medicinal tonic soup. Astragalus soups are very pleasant-tasting, since astragalus has a mild, slightly sweet flavor. Put a few slices of the root into a pot of soup and simmer for awhile. The longer the soup is simmered, the more benefit from the astragalus. When the soup is done, remove the root slices since they are too tough to eat. This is an excellent way to help family members get through the cold and flu season without getting sick. They won't even suspect that astragalus has been added to the soup. In Oriental medicine, astragalus root is said to stimulate the *wei chi* or protective energy; roughly what we would call the immunity. Astragalus is also superb as an ingredient in cough syrup.

Astragalus is most commonly sold in thin slices of the dried taproot. Extracts, tinctures and encapsulated astragalus products are also widely available. Astragalus roots can be found in any Chinatown or in your local natural food store.

In one of the most impressive studies done with astragalus, researchers at the University of Texas Medical Center in Houston found that astragalus extracts could completely restore the function of compromised immune cells taken from the blood of human cancer patients. This stellar research showed that when damaged immune cells were stimulated by astragalus, they could equal and even surpass the function of cells from healthy humans. Another Chinese study showed that frequency and duration of the common cold could be reduced from 4.6 days to an average of 2.6 days. At the National Cancer Institute, astragalus was found to restore the immune system in 90 percent of cancer patients.

Five to fifteen grams per day of the herb is an average dose, and a decoction is the recommended preparation method. Chewing on a piece of the root is soothing for a sore throat due to the high content of polysaccharides and mucilage. Further tests have shown its normalizing effect on the nervous, hormonal and immune systems.

For people who catch colds easily and frequently, have shortness of breath, weak lungs and low energy, this is an excellent herb. A great boon to those who are convalescing, astragalus benefits malnutrition and diarrhea, increases appetite, strengthens digestion, treats exhaustion, helps poorly healing sores and ulcerations. Astragalus has no known toxicity and can be used to lessen the side effects of chemotherapy and radiation and inhibit the growth of tumors.

Black Cohosh   *(Cimicifuga racemosa)*
Part used: Root
Actions: Emmenagogue, antispasmodic, sedative, alterative, nervine, tonic, antitussive, diuretic, diaphoretic, antirheumatic, oxytocic, peripheral vasodilator, anti-inflammatory, sedative, hypotensive
Indications: This native American herb has a reputation as a powerful antispasmodic, relaxant and analgesic. Black cohosh is indicated when there is dull aching heaviness in the limbs and congestion and rheumatoid-like conditions, including fibromyalgia. It is often tremendously helpful for neck and back pains.

Commonly used as a normalizer of the female reproductive system, it is especially useful in painful cramping conditions. It has been hailed as a primary herb in formulations for menopause. The archetype of black cohosh is: severe cramping, heavy menstrual flow with low back pains and heaviness in the thighs. It works well in combination with black haw *(Viburnum prunifolium)* or crampbark *(Viburnum opulus)*.

As an antispasmodic, it eases pulmonary complaints

such as whooping cough, asthma and bronchitis. Its sedative properties may help those who can't sleep well due to aches and pains or headache.

In Boerike's homeopathic *Materia Medica,* black cohosh is indicated for great depression and a sensation of being enveloped by a black cloud. In other homeopathic literature it is used when a person is melancholy, gloomy, irritable and despondent and in a state of dark hopelessness. One hundred years ago, homeopaths used herbs in tincture doses, making this information as relevant today as it was then.

Contraindications: Black cohosh is contraindicated in pregnancy and for those with low blood pressure. Do not exceed 2 teaspoons of tincture over the course of a 24-hour period. Excessive amounts of black cohosh can result in nausea, vomiting, frontal headaches or headaches behind the eyes, dizziness and convulsions.

Black Walnut (*Juglans nigra*)

Part used: Hulls and leaves

Actions: Anthelmintic, vermifuge, antifungal, astringent, alterative, antiseptic, antimicrobial

Indications: Black walnut hull and leaf have strong antifungal properties, making them useful for healing fungal conditions such as ringworm, athlete's foot, fingernail and toenail fungus and other fungal conditions of the skin as well as herpes and eczema. A compress can be made by saturating a cloth in the freshly simmered decoction, and applying topically.

As an anthelmintic, black walnut expels worms and parasites. It is also effective for treating candidiasis in 1 teaspoon (5 ml) doses, given three times a day. Studies begun at the University of Missouri demonstrated that black walnuts contain alkaloids which show anticancer properties. Juglone contained within the leaves and hulls is antimicrobial.

Black walnut hulls turn black and spoil quickly once they have fallen from the tree in autumn. Tincture made from the green hulls is reputed to be the most beneficial. Wear rubber gloves when cutting the hulls from the nut as they stain the skin dark brown for more than a week, making them a valuable ingredient in self-tanning suntan lotions. Encapsulated black walnut products are also available.

Burdock   *(Arctium lappa)*
Part used: Roots and seeds
Actions: Alterative, diuretic, diaphoretic, antirheumatic, antiseptic, tonic, demulcent, hepatic, antimicrobial, nutritive, lymphatic, aperient
Indications: This large biennial is widely used as a powerful blood purifier and alterative for chronic skin eruptions such as acne, psoriasis and eczema. It is helpful for styes, boils, skin rashes and canker sores. It is even more effective when combined with yellow dock, sarsaparilla and milk thistle. It is excellent applied topically as a poultice or compress and internally, drunk as a tea. To make the tea, place 1 teaspoon of dried root in 1 cup of cold water. Bring to a boil and simmer for 20 minutes. Drink twice a day.

As an antirheumatic, burdock is beneficial for arthritis, gout and inflammations. According to a pharmacognostic study done in 1958, burdock contains bactericidal and fungicidal constituents which inhibit *staphylococcus aureus.* Burdock contains a polysaccharide called inulin, which strengthens the liver, spleen and pancreas and helps regulate blood sugar metabolism. Inulin is a superb immune modulator which binds to white blood cells enhancing their activity. In a study at Nagoya University in 1984, Japanese scientists discovered a substance in burdock which has the capacity to reduce cell mutation. This substance was called the B-factor. Burdock is one of the primary ingredients in Essiac, an herbal formula reputed to heal cancer patients.

Burdock is also famous as a lymphatic cleanser and kidney tonic. The seeds are an effective diuretic for edema. Its diuretic action helps the kidneys to clear harmful acids from the blood, thus reducing fluid retention. As a mild bitter, burdock helps improve digestion.

Although burdock is effective as a bitter, its taste is not bitter. It has a rather mild and nutty flavor, somewhat like an earthy carrot without the sweetness, although some say it tastes like a blend of celery and potato. In Japan it is called gobo, and is highly prized as both a vegetable and medicinal herb. My friend, Toshiko, an extraordinary Japanese cook and director of a shiatsu school in Vermont, taught me to make this delicious dish with burdock:

Toshiko's Burdock-Carrot Sauté

2-3 fresh burdock roots, scrubbed clean and sliced julienne

Dark, toasted sesame oil for cooking

3-4 carrots, cleaned and sliced julienne

Tamari or soy sauce to taste

1 large onion sliced in half and then in crescents

1-2 tablespoons sesame seeds, toasted in a dry skillet

Steam the burdock roots until crisp-tender. Sauté steamed burdock roots in the oil until nearly cooked through; then add carrots and onions and cook until crisp-tender. Add sesame seeds and heat through. Season with tamari.

Cat's Claw   (Uncaria tomentosa)
Part used: Root and inner bark
Actions: Antiviral, antiulcer, antioxidant, antiallergic, anti-inflammatory, antiarthritic, antiseptic, hypotensive, sedative, vasodilator, antiasthmatic, antitumor

Indications: Since the early 1990's, cat's claw has been in the news as a veritable panacea for nearly every degenerative disease. For hundreds of years, Peruvian Indian tribes have harvested the root and inner bark of this climbing woody vine for an impressive list of ailments. Growing over 100 feet in length and reaching a circumference of nearly 12 inches, cat's claw has sharp, curved thorns, much like the claws of a cat or jaguar. Since its arrival in the United States several years ago, cat's claw has been used for arthritis, tumors, digestive disorders, lupus, fibromyalgia, diabetes, chronic fatigue, chemical and environmental allergies, respiratory infections, candidiasis, Crohn's disease, hemorrhoids and to counter the side effects of chemotherapy and radiation.

Austrian physician Klaus Keplinger has reported his observations showing cat's claw's effectiveness in benefiting those with shingles, multiple sclerosis and even AIDS. Italian studies show that certain compounds in cat's claw called quinovic acid glycosides exhibit antiviral properties, and other compounds in the plant possess anti-inflammatory, antiallergic, adaptogenic, antiulcer and antitumor properties and enhance T-cell activity.

Because of the flurry of interest in cat's claw in the U.S. and limited supplies of the herb, the quality of cat's claw products can vary considerably. Only the inner bark and root have medicinal value, but some Peruvian sources of cat's claw have been found to contain outer bark, twigs, stems and inner wood of the vine. Another problem is that more than 20 different indigenous Peruvian herbs are commonly referred to as "uña de gato," and some of these are toxic. Only *U. tomentosa* and *U. guianensis* have been shown to have medicinal value.

Scientist Keplinger believes that preparations made by traditional methods that involve cooking the herb are best. Make a decoction by cooking approximately 1 cup of shredded bark in 1 quart of water. Simmer slowly for 45 minutes. Cool for 10 minutes and strain. Add enough water to make one quart. Keep refrigerated. The suggested dose is 2 ounces mixed with warm water, taken once daily on an empty stomach.

Cleavers   *(Galium aparine)*
Part used: Whole herb
Actions: Diuretic, aperient, lymphatic, tonic, alterative, astringent, anti-inflammatory, hypotensive, antibiotic
Indications: Cleavers is highly esteemed as a lymph system tonic. It is effective against chronic inflammatory conditions, including psoriasis, eczema, arthritis and swollen lymph nodes. It is excellent in the treatment of chronic fatigue syndrome. It is useful in tonsillitis and adenoid conditions. It has a long history of use in the treatment of ulcers, especially in combination with demulcents, and in the treatment of tumors. Its diuretic effects make it a safe and useful tonic in cystitis.

It is most effective as a fresh plant juice or succus, 1 to 2 ounces taken up to four times per day, or as a liquid extract, taken in ½-teaspoon to 1-teaspoon (2-½ to 5 ml) doses. An infusion of cleavers is best used for urinary problems such as cystitis and for reducing fevers. A cloth dipped in the infusion and wrung out can be applied topically as a compress on burns and itchy or inflamed skin conditions. The infusion can also be used as a hair rinse for dandruff. The infusion of cleavers is made by pouring 8 ounces of boiling water over 3 teaspoons of freshly dried herb and steeping 15 minutes. Because cleavers contains up to 90 percent water, many herbalists suggest drying it prior to preparation.

In *The Scientific Validation of Herbal Medicine,* Daniel B. Mowrey suggests combining cleavers with uva ursi and buchu for maximum benefit for acute urinary tract inflammation. Eclectic physicians used it for eliminating kidney stones and gallstones. Cleavers shows hypotensive activity, making it useful in the treatment of heart disease.

Devil's Claw   *(Harpagophytum procumbens)*
Part used: Rhizome
Actions: Anti-inflammatory, anodyne, antirheumatic, hepatic, analgesic, sedative, diuretic
Indications: Known for its anti-inflammatory effects, this desert plant has been valuable in the treatment of some types of arthritis. As with many botanicals, it is best used as a whole plant extract. In *The Holistic Herbal,* David Hoffmann recommends taking 1 to 2 mls (about ¼ to ½ teaspoon) of the tincture three times per day.

In Africa, the infusion is traditionally used for blood disorders, fevers, indigestion and as a bitter tonic. The fresh tuber is made into a salve for boils, ulcers and skin lesions. The extract has been used for allergic reactions, headache and pain, as well as for diseases of the liver, kidney and bladder. Dr. Rudolf Fritz Weiss recommends the use of devil's claw in dyspepsia and gall bladder disease, but because of its strong bitter properties, cautions against it for stomach ulcers. He also suggests its benefit for older patients with rheumatic complaints, obesity and high blood lipids, since German research shows that it lowers cholesterol.

Devil's Club   *(Oplopanax horridum)*
Part used: Root
Actions: Expectorant, respiratory stimulant, hypoglycemic
Indications: Commonly used for the treatment of blood sugar disorders, devil's club is also a safe stimulating expectorant which helps with loosening mucous in chest colds and bronchitis. Michael Moore writes that as either a cold infusion or a tincture, it can help with rheumatoid arthritis and some autoimmune disorders.

According to its long history of use for adult-onset, insulin-resistant diabetes, it shows clear benefits. Moore observes that it seems to work best for stocky, middle-aged people with elevated blood lipids, high blood pressure and early signs of adult-onset diabetes. Besides aiding stress and providing a sense of well-being, it helps lessen appetite in those who are trying to lose weight and decreases the desire for sugary foods. An amphoteric herb, devil's club has value for those who are either hypoglycemic or hyperglycemic in that it raises blood sugar levels that are too low and lowers those which are too high. It allows insulin to be present longer in the body. For Type I diabetics (those whose bodies don't produce insulin), devil's club is not effective. For a 150-pound person who is not taking insulin, an average dose might be 1 teaspoon (5 ml) of the tincture, two to three times per day. Those with low blood sugar may achieve better results by taking 1 teaspoon (5 ml) in the morning and repeating that dose in the evening.

Echinacea *(Echinacea spp.)*

Part used: Root and herb

Actions: Antibacterial, antiviral, antimicrobial, vulnerary, alterative, adaptogenic, immunostimulant, antifungal, anti-inflammatory

Indications: Considered number-one in a list of the top 10 herbs in America today, echinacea is a safe, nontoxic immune-enhancing herb. Extensive clinical studies show that this North American herb stimulates the surface or secretory immune system and works best as a protective agent against pathogenic (virus, bacteria, candida) invasion or overgrowth. For deep immune imbalances, echinacea can be combined with more tonic or deep immune herbs such as reishi, astragalus, Siberian ginseng or ligustrum.

As an alterative it has been used for virtually every disease of the immune system. One of the best blood purifiers, it is especially beneficial for infections and inflammations. It increases the proliferation of stem cells in both the bone marrow and lymphatic tissue, where immune cells are produced. It also increases the number and activity of these immunocompetent cells in the blood and lymph systems. Some of the documented research on echinacea shows that it promotes blood clotting in wound healing and it works better than cortisone in keeping infections localized. It increases leukocyte production in bone marrow in radiology patients and it is an effective antibiotic against bacterial infections, including *Streptococcus* and *Staphylococcus*. Echinacea protects cells against viral infections including herpes, canker sores and influenza and may have tumor-inhibiting capabilities.

Recent German research indicates that in a comparison of three commonly used echinacea species (*E. angustifolia, E. pallida* and *E. purpurea), E. purpurea* appeared to have the strongest action. Most authorities and American herbals of the 20th century usually claim that *E. angustifolia* is the best one to use. The German study is interesting since, with the growing popularity of echinacea, several wild species, including *E. angustifolia,* are becoming threatened.

E. purpurea is the easiest to grow, and the market supply of it comes from cultivated, rather than wild-harvested plants. If you buy *E. purpurea,* you are helping to prevent the depletion of echinacea in the wild. In addition, *E. purpurea* shows slightly more phagocytosis (the destruction of bacteria and foreign bodies by macrophages) than either *E. pallida* or *E. angustifolia.* Steven Foster, long considered one of the U.S. authorities on echinacea, believes that *E. purpurea* is unequivocally the best species to use.

It is the isobutylamides, primary components of echinacea, that cause the tingling or numbing sensation on the tongue. Some experts claim that one of the best ways to determine the quality of an echinacea root is to taste it. If it causes a ''buzzing'' or tingling sensation, it is of good quality. Today, some of the echinacea sold commercially is actually adulterated with *parthenium integrifolium,* an herb in the aster family called prairie dock or Missouri snakeroot, which has different actions from echinacea.

Echinacea works well in either teas or tinctures, but one of the active constituents, isobutylamides, is only soluble in alcohol. Although the root is most commonly used, effective preparations can be made which include seeds, flowers and leaves. Two teaspoons of the tincture every one to two hours for five days at the earliest stage of infection is an effective dose. Some people find they get better results by using the following shotgun approach when they feel a cold coming on: One hour before bed, take one ½ ounce of echinacea tincture. Then, just before bed, take another ½ ounce. Proponents claim that by morning, their cold symptoms are just a memory.

Elecampane   *(Inula helenium)*
Part used: Root
Actions: Expectorant, antimicrobial, diaphoretic, diuretic, alterative, tonic, anthelmintic, antibacterial, antitussive, anti-inflammatory
Indications: Long used as a safe tonic herb, this stimulating expectorant is a specific for bronchial coughs, especially in children and in the elderly. Whenever there is copious sticky mucus in the lungs, with a chronic, wet, rattling cough, as in bronchitis or emphysema, elecampane is indicated. Once a specific for tuberculosis, this striking, yellow-flowered plant is an excellent decongestant.

It is a bitter, aromatic tonic which increases appetite, promotes digestion and increases sweating, making it a good choice for those recuperating from the flu. Useful for chronic inflammatory conditions, elecampane may also be helpful for ulcerated colon, cystitis and night sweats. It is contraindicated for hot, dry coughs.

Since inulin, contained in the root, influences blood sugar, it is not recommended for diabetics. Alantolactone, another compound in the plant, helps expel intestinal parasites. The bitter, camphor-like flavor of elecampane makes it much more palatable in tincture form than in a tea. Make the tincture of the freshly dried root in 75 percent grain alcohol using 1 part herb to 5 parts grain alcohol.

Garlic   (*Allium sativum*)
Part used: Bulb
Actions: Antibiotic, expectorant, antifungal, antiparasitic, antiprotozoan, diaphoretic, hypotensive, antithrombotic, antidiabetic, alterative, tonic, antiseptic, antispasmodic, anthelmintic, stimulant, anticarcinogenic, cardioprotective
Indications: One of the most thoroughly studied of all medicinal plants, garlic has been used throughout the ages for everything from gangrene and leprosy to warding off the bubonic plague. Often called "the stinking rose," garlic is the world's second oldest medicine after ephedra.

Considered superior for treating many respiratory ailments, including whooping cough, bronchitis, coughs and colds, its antibiotic effects are largely due to the action of a compound called allicin. Allicin also acts against *Candida albicans, Trichomonas, Staphylococcus, E. coli, Salmonella* and *Shigella.* Garlic came to be called Russian penicillin during World War I for its effectiveness against battle wounds and dysentery. Garlic's antimicrobial action benefits chronic infections, especially those of the lungs and respiratory system.

As a cardiovascular remedy, garlic is superb, reducing blood pressure, decreasing harmful LDL cholesterol levels and lowering the platelet aggregation that can lead to strokes and heart attacks.

The antihepatotoxic properties of garlic protect the liver against toxins such as lead, mercury and heavy metal poisoning. It is a powerful free-radical scavenger, retarding aging, arthritis and cancer. Its antioxidant effect makes it a beneficial adjunct to radiation or chemotherapy by reducing damage done to normal tissue by these therapies. It, like echinacea, increases phagocytosis and has tumor-inhibiting capabilities. An article on the therapeutic benefits of garlic in the *Journal of the American Medical Association*, states, "No other substance, either natural or synthetic, can match garlic's proven therapeutic effectiveness."

As an antifungal, garlic has been shown effective in treating the fungi that cause athlete's foot, fingernail and toenail fungus and vaginal as well as systemic yeast infections.

To garner these benefits, a therapeutic dose of garlic is 18 mg of garlic oil, 9 grams of fresh garlic, or 1 to 2 large cloves daily. Recent research shows that garlic is just as effective raw, cooked or deodorized. If the smell of garlic makes you turn up your nose, try chewing on cloves or parsley as a breath freshener after a meal of garlic. Since cooked garlic is less odiferous than fresh, try roasting a garlic bulb. Slice ½ inch off the top of the garlic bulb, drizzle a little olive oil over it and place in an oven-proof dish or wrap tightly in heavy-duty foil. Roast at 300 degrees for about forty minutes or until very tender. Spread on toasted bread or include in savory dishes.

I have found the following recipe to be a very effective (and tasty) formula for sore throat and respiratory congestion.

Sweet Garlic Honey

    13 or more garlic cloves, crushed
    Juice of one lemon
    3–4 whole cloves

3–5 drops of peppermint essential oil
8 ounces honey

Place all ingredients in a pint jar and cover with honey. Keep refrigerated. Steep four to six weeks. Strain and use as a sweetener in your tea or as a powerful cough syrup. The preservative properties of honey give this a long shelf life.

Ginger   *(Zingiber officinale)*
Part used: Root (rhizome)
Actions: Diaphoretic, carminative, rubefacient, stimulant, anti-inflammatory, antispasmodic, emmenagogue, anti-emetic, antitussive
Indications: Almost a panacea, ginger seems to be making the news lately with ever more uses for this common household herb. Dr. James Duke says that research indicates that 1/30th of an ounce of powdered ginger is more potent against motion sickness in some people than 50 to 100 mg of Dramamine. It is quite possible that a 12-ounce bottle of ginger ale may be more effective in preventing motion sickness in some people than 50 to 100 mg of Dramamine. Both the fresh and dried rhizome have been shown to prevent motion sickness and suppress vomiting. Ginger is often taken in capsule form and, unlike Dramamine, does not cause drowsiness.

Generally regarded as safe for everyone—from children to the elderly—ginger's warming qualities make it an important addition to respiratory, digestive and circulatory formulas. Because it acts as an adjuvent or catalyst in combination with other herbs, it is often added to formulas to activate or enhance their effectiveness.

As a digestive aid, ginger helps to relieve flatulence, bloating and digestive distress. Ginger also helps to promote good circulation and alleviate cramping. For those with cold hands and feet, ginger helps to bring the circulation to the periphery. For both digestive and menstrual cramping, ginger brings relief with its antispasmodic action. It has also been used as a treatment for ulcers. Certain aromatic compounds in ginger called *gingerols* have been cited for their anti-inflammatory effects in treating rheumatoid arthritis.

I have used the following formula dozens of times for nausea, gastric complaints and cramping. It is simple, delicious and the syrup stores for about two weeks in the refrigerator. Thanks to herbalist Kate Gilday for this recipe:

Kate's Homemade Ginger Ale
    2 cups fresh ginger root, chopped
    ½ cup maple syrup
    1 quart spring water
    Perrier or sparkling mineral water

Simmer the ginger root in spring water for one-half hour. Strain out the ginger root and compost the root. Add the maple syrup to the ginger root decoction. It is strong! To make ginger ale, add 1 to 3 tablespoons of this ginger syrup to 8 ounces of sparkling water. If you are lucky enough to have access to maple sap (not syrup) during the spring sugaring season, add the sap in place of the spring water for added nutrients and a delicious treat.

Ginkgo   (Ginkgo biloba)
Part used: Leaf
Actions: Vasodilator, anti-inflammatory, antiasthmatic
Indications: Considered the oldest living tree species on earth, ginkgo survived by being protected in the Chinese monasteries. It is the only surviving tree of its genus. One of the most extensively researched herbs, ginkgo has been shown to have a profound effect on cerebral function and circulation as well as on many vascular disorders. It may

be beneficial for many diseases associated with aging such as memory loss, heart disease, stroke, impotence and some forms of deafness and blindness.

Research shows that ginkgo has the ability to prevent blood clotting in strokes and heart attacks, asthma attacks and organ graft rejection. Ginkgo can alleviate intermittent claudication (pain, cramping and weakness in the legs due to cholesterol deposits in the arteries) by improving blood flow to the legs and calves. Ginkgo also thins the blood, thereby preventing clotting and benefiting those with atherosclerosis. Ginkgo has also proven effective against tinnitus (ringing the ears) and vertigo (dizziness).

Ginkgo's clinical effects are largely due to its ability to dilate blood vessels and increase circulation to the head, heart and extremities. If the conditions mentioned above are due to impaired circulation, ginkgo can be of help.

Ginkgo extracts also show great promise in the treatment of senility, dementia and early stages of Alzheimer's disease. The effective dose for treating Alzheimer's disease in one study was 80 mg three times daily. The dose most often recommended is 120 mg daily. For those with memory loss and other signs of dementia, the effects of ginkgo are most evident after two or more months of continual use. The leaf extract is considered one of the best ways to use ginkgo, although many feel that the concentrated standardized extract (in capsule form) containing 24 percent flavone glycosides is the most effective. Two to six capsules daily is the suggested dose.

Although generally recognized as safe, if dizziness or headaches occur in elderly persons taking 240 mg daily, decrease the dose to 120 mg daily and slowly increase to 240 mg over the course of six to eight weeks. Some sources say that ginkgo is contraindicated for those with blood clotting disorders and, in extremely large doses, irritability, restlessness, vomiting and diarrhea have been reported. However, current reviews of ginkgo's safety concur that ginkgo biloba leaf or leaf extract is safe and does not pose a hazard.

Ginseng *(Panax ginseng, P. quinquefolius, and Eleutherococcus senticosus)*

Part used: Root

Actions: Tonic, stimulant, adaptogen, hypoglycemic, immunomodulator, rejuvenative

Indications: Nearly everyone has heard of the seemingly mystical, magical and curative properties of ginseng. Purported to be an elixir of longevity, a tonic for enhancing sexual performance, a stress-buster and energy booster as well as a panacea for many other ailments, ginseng has become so popular that it is now available for sale in vials and capsules on the countertops of convenience stores nationwide. Whether these ginseng vials or ginseng "pep" pills contain enough ginseng to be effective is questionable. Because ginseng is rare and expensive, it has often been adulterated. One study shows that more than half of the ginseng products evaluated contained so little ginseng as to have no effect.

Long esteemed in the Orient for its tonic effects, Asian ginseng *(P. ginseng)* is available in both red and white forms. Red ginseng is steamed and dried, making it more stimulating and useful for older people with low energy and weak vitality. White ginseng refers to the peeled, dried root of Asian ginseng. The white variety (actually a pale yellow in color) is cooler, often combined with other herbs and more useful for those who need an energy boost. White ginseng benefits the lungs and digestive system. American ginseng *(P. quinquefolius)* is a tonic with a long history of Native American use for fevers, headaches, dysentery and as a fertility tonic. It is considered so valuable to the Chinese that literally tons of wild American ginseng have been exported to the Orient annually since colonial times, pushing it to the edge of extinction and leading to its threatened or endangered status in more than half of the 50 states. Because it can fetch up to $600 per pound, the young immature roots of American ginseng continue to be harvested illegally. Buy only ginseng which is woods-grown, not wildcrafted.

Reputed to be a men's tonic, ginseng is beneficial to both men and women. Christopher Hobbs writes in *The Ginsengs* that it can improve physical as well as mental performance under stress, improve reaction time, prolong life and combat senility. In China it is used to treat heart disease and cancer. A 1990 study showed that 100 mg of standardized ginseng extract increased immune cells, including T-cell counts. Ginsenosides (saponin compounds in the plant) have been found to stimulate bone marrow production, stimulate the immune system, inhibit tumor growth, stabilize blood pressure, detoxify the liver and balance blood sugar. Although hailed as an aphrodisiac and male virility tonic, research is inconclusive as to whether ginseng has an effect on sex hormones.

Panax ginseng is generally regarded as a safe herb, providing protection against mental and physical fatigue, nonspecific resistance to stress and supporting adrenal gland function. Perhaps its reputation as a panacea is due to its ability to restore strength, balance and harmony so that the body can heal itself.

Experts advise that to err on the safe side, don't use ginseng if you have high blood pressure, headaches, insomnia, inflammation, asthma, heart palpitations or infections associated with high fever. Pregnant women should avoid ginseng because of its hormonal interactions, and ginseng is not considered safe for children.

Ginseng can be taken in several ways. An excellent and cost-effective way is to use a ginseng cooker, which slowly cooks the root, producing a concentrated water extract. To make ginseng tea, simmer 3 teaspoons of the dried or sliced root in 8 ounces water, covered, for 45 minutes. Strain and drink one cup two or three times daily. A suggested dose for ginseng tincture is ½ teaspoon (2-½ mls) in warm water two to three times a day. Better results are seen by taking this dose for a month or two. Then take a break for a week and continue for another one to two months. Standardized ginseng products which guarantee 4 to 5 percent ginsenosides are considered best. The recommended dose is usually 100 mg one or two times daily. Since the effectiveness of ginsenosides diminish over time, use the capsules or tablets within a year of purchase.

Siberian ginseng or Eleuthero *(Eleutherococcus senticosus)* is not a true ginseng at all but has similar characteristics and deserves mention here. It is best known as a safe, adaptogenic tonic which is one of the most thoroughly studied of the adaptogens. Less expensive than *panax* ginseng, eleuthero has been shown to increase stamina and work capacity among factory workers and boost performance levels of athletes as well as reduce recovery rates. It is frequently given to the elderly and those recovering from chronic illness as it improves energy and vitality while benefiting circulation and edema. It helps depression by increasing the availability of seratonin in the brain. One of the greatest benefits of Siberian ginseng is in helping people cope with stress.

Even though Siberian ginseng doesn't have a direct effect on cancer cells, it can increase immune resistance and reduce side effects resulting from radiation and chemotherapy. Researchers found that residents of cold regions of China got fewer colds and cases of bronchitis when they regularly took Siberian ginseng. Eleuthero, like panax ginseng, lessens fatigue, stabilizes blood sugar and alleviates depression.

A standard dose of Siberian ginseng is 3 cups per day of decoction or 30 drops of tincture one to three times a day or 2 capsules, one to three times daily. Considered very safe, Siberian ginseng seems to work best if used as a tonic over the course of a three-month period, but it is safe to take for nine months or longer.

Goldenseal *(Hydrastis canadensis)*
Part used: Root
Actions: Antibiotic, antimicrobial, anti-inflammatory, immune stimulant, bitter tonic, astringent, antiseptic, laxative, diuretic, alterative, hemostatic
Indications: Like ginseng, goldenseal's soaring popularity has caused its near extinction. Even rarer than ginseng, with over 150,000 pounds of it consumed in the United States alone, goldenseal should never be harvested from the wild, and only cultivated goldenseal should be purchased. Because of its scarcity (goldenseal was considered rare as far back as 75 years ago), goldenseal has often been adulterated with turmeric and even bloodroot, another endangered plant.

This powerful, antimicrobial herb is now sadly misused and overused. It has a reputation among most Americans today as an "herbal antibiotic" in combination with echinacea for colds and flu. However, recent clinical research shows that one of goldenseal's active constituents, berberine, is poorly absorbed in the small intestine, indicating that even 26 capsules of goldenseal powder would not provide enough berberine to act as a systemic antibiotic. In fact, taking goldenseal at the first signs of a cold can have the negative effects of injuring the stomach and intestinal function, inhibiting the body's natural defenses and weakening the immune response, thereby prolonging the illness.

The tragedy is that the majority of people who buy goldenseal in the United States are both wasting their money and further endangering this nearly extinct plant. In his excellent article on goldenseal in the winter 1996–1997 issue of *Medical Herbalism,* Editor Paul Bergner writes, "Taking goldenseal or berberine internally will not directly kill or inhibit bacteria or other infectious agents in most of these conditions, (colds or flu) "unless coming in direct contact with the infected tissue."

Goldenseal works by both toning and increasing secretions in the mucous membranes. This makes goldenseal (as well as other herbs containing berberine) beneficial for acute and chronic mucous membrane conditions. Since berberine is excreted through the urine, goldenseal may act as an effective antibiotic in cystitis and urinary tract infections.

To use goldenseal topically for an eye infection, make a tea by steeping ¼ teaspoon of goldenseal powder in ½ cup of just-boiled water for 15 to 20 minutes. Once cooled to body temperature, strain the tea through a coffee filter. Then, using an eyedropper, put one drop in the infected eye. By morning, the infection may be completely cleared.

Many goldenseal substitutes are readily available, most of them more abundant than goldenseal and some, such as goldthread (*coptis*), contain even more berberine than goldenseal. A common woodland plant of the eastern United States, goldthread is useful for stomach complaints, canker sores, fevers and infections. Some analogs for goldenseal include the ubiquitous barberry (*berberis*), which grows prolifically throughout the New England woodlands and is cultivated as a common landscape shrub. Barberry is an effective remedy for cystitis, bronchitis, second-stage bacterial infections, abscessed teeth and ear infections. Some herbalists consider it to be more effective than echinacea for well-established colds. Barberry contains at least seven alkaloids in addition to berberine.

Oregon grape root (*Berberis/Mahonia aquifolium*) can be used in place of goldenseal, especially in digestive complaints, chronic skin conditions and mucous membrane problems. A traditional desert herb, yerba mansa (*Anemopsis californica*) is a popular replacement for goldenseal in the Southwest. Although it does not contain berberine or related alkaloids, it works well as a mucous membrane remedy.

In the Southeast, yellowroot (*Xanthorhiza simplicissima*) is a popular folk remedy which is used interchangeably with goldenseal and is far less threatened.

Still, for secondary stages of bronchitis and bacterial infection, goldenseal achieves the quickest results. I use goldenseal as if it were pure gold, reserving it only for conditions in which it is indicated and using it conservatively. The goldenseal powder I have carried in my first aid kit for nearly five years is still as effective as it was when I purchased it. Goldenseal's powerful constituents insure its long shelf life—beyond that of most herbs.

A remarkable immunostimulant and activator of macrophages, goldenseal destroys harmful pathogens such as bacteria, fungi, viruses and tumor cells. In vitro, goldenseal is effective against a whole swath of microorganisms including *E. coli, Giardia lamblia, Staphylococcus aureus, Streptococcus pyrogenes, Salmonella paratyphi* and *Candida albicans*. Some other uses of goldenseal and its analogs include tonsillitis, skin eruptions, gum disease and ringworm.

The extremely bitter taste of goldenseal makes it much more appealing in tinctures or capsules. The recommended dose is ¼ teaspoon of the tincture or 1 or 2 capsules three times daily. In spite of its potent compounds, goldenseal's only potential toxicity is to pregnant women because of its berberine content.

Grapefruit Seed Extract
Part used: Extract of the seed
Actions: Antimicrobial, antiparasitic, antibiotic, antifungal, antiviral, antibacterial
Indications: A powerful concentrate extracted from grapefruit and other citrus seeds, grapefruit seed extract destroys

bacteria, fungi, yeast, mold, viruses, parasites and other pathogens on contact. Originally developed as a natural fungicide to protect fruits and vegetables during shipping, this bitter-tasting extract has made its way into the health food market as a supplement. Available in the form of capsules of liquid extracts, some of the common brand names for this product are Nutribiotic, Proseed and Citricidal. Grapefruit seed extract is nontoxic in dilute solution but must never be used full strength. In laboratory tests, it has been shown to be effective against a wide variety of pathogens such as *E. coli, Salmonella spp., Staphylococcus spp., Candida albicans, Aspergillus spp., Entamoeba histolytica,* herpes simplex virus, type 1, influenza A2 virus and *Giardia lamblia.*

It is this last parasite, *Giardia,* that often contaminates mountain streams and other water sources of campers and hikers. Grapefruit seed extract can be added to drinking water to prevent this problem as well as traveler's diarrhea. One company makes a product called "Traveler's Friend," for this very purpose. Dilute solutions of the extract can be used for skin ailments, athlete's foot, fungal and yeast infections and gargle for sore throats. Advocates suggest using a few drops mixed into 8 ounces of water as a douche for vaginal infections and adding 3 or 4 drops to a small glass of water as an oral rinse for gingivitis and gum disease. In a spray bottle, combined with essential oils of chamomile and tea tree, grapefruit seed extract can promote healing of poison ivy rash, cold sores and fever blisters. CJ Puotinen recommends adding ⅛ teaspoon of grapefruit seed extract to the water reservoir of your humidifier once a week and adding a few drops daily thereafter, as a disinfectant.

Licorice   (*Glycyrrhiza glabra*)
Part used: Root
Actions: Demulcent, anti-inflammatory, expectorant, antitussive, antiviral, hepatoprotectant, adrenal tonic, laxative.

Indications: A perennial herb of the pea family, licorice root's sweet, aromatic flavor is known to almost everyone in the form of black candies, but today licorice candy is usually sweetened with anise. A compound in licorice, glycyrrhizin, makes it 50 to 100 times sweeter than cane sugar.

Licorice is a time-honored herbal medicine throughout the world. It is used for gastric, peptic and duodenal ulcers and has a soothing effect on the digestive tract. An Irish study found licorice extract to relieve ulcer symptoms more effectively than the popular ulcer medication, Tagamet. Licorice has been included in Chinese herbal formulas for centuries, where it is considered a great detoxifier and harmonizing ingredient in complex formulas. In Japan, clinical trials using licorice for chronic hepatitis have been so successful that glycyrrhizin is now a standard medical treatment there.

Licorice is a soothing decongestant for acute respiratory problems, including coughs, bronchitis and sore throats. It has the ability to control blood sugar and has hormonal balancing effects. Its potent antiviral properties are useful for treating influenza and the herpes virus, in addition to canker sores and cold sores.

Licorice is also an important liver herb comparable to milk thistle. In fact, milk thistle and licorice work exceptionally well in tandem for treating liver ailments such as chronic active hepatitis. Several *in vitro* trials illustrate glycyrrhizin's ability to protect liver cells from damage from a variety of chemical agents. In addition, glycyrrhizin stimulates the immune system, activates macrophages and enhances natural killer T-cell activity.

Licorice has many of the same effects as cortisol in reducing inflammation. This makes it beneficial for conditions like arthritis, asthma, bowel disease, psoriasis and eczema by inhibiting the body's inflammatory response. Studies also show that licorice derivatives are as effective topically as hydrocortisone for many skin ailments including dermatitis, impetigo, hemorrhoids and herpes.

Although licorice does not suppress the immune system in the same way that steroids do, both pharmaceutical cortisone and the glycyrrhizin compound in licorice may cause fluid retention, weight gain, sodium retention, low blood potassium, weakness (due to low potassium) and sometimes headache. Licorice should be avoided by pregnant women and those with high blood pressure, history of heart disease, stroke, diabetes and glaucoma.

Deglycyrrhinized licorice products (those which have been treated to remove the glycyrrhizin) have long been used in Europe and are now available in the United States and Canada, While a cup of licorice root tea daily is considered safe, more than five cups of strongly brewed licorice tea per day or long-term use of lower doses could cause side effects. Glycyrrhizin is unsafe at daily doses of 0.5 g, equivalent to 5,000 mg of herb per day. Elderly persons who may be on other medications and whose metabolism is slower, should be cautious about using licorice.

Lomatium (*Lomatium dissectum*)

Part used: Root

Actions: Antiviral, immunostimulant, expectorant

Indications: A native of rocky areas in the western United States, lomatium has been used as a medicine for centuries by native Americans, herbalists and naturopathic physicians. Although it is not well-known in the rest of the country, in the Western states, it is used in the treatment of viral conditions, lung problems, pneumonia and severe fevers.

Besides benefiting simple head colds, its most promising use is in the treatment of chronic fatigue syndrome and respiratory virus infections. Its aromatic resins act as an expectorant in respiratory conditions, and as a mild immune stimulant it may be a helpful adjunct in the treatment of HIV. Herbalist Deb Soule uses lomatium in her immune response-stimulating formula. She suggests using a combination of equal parts lomatium, usnea, echinacea root and goldenseal root for seven to ten days for conditions such as bronchitis, pneumonia, flus, candida, colds, skin lesions and as part of a protocol for HIV, herpes and chronic fatigue syndrome.

Some of the compounds in lomatium have demonstrated their ability to stimulate the rate of phagocytosis (the devouring of foreign bodies by immune cells). Lomatium can greatly reduce the occurrence of respiratory infections in those with Epstein-Barr and cytomegalovirus. Some people have experienced skin rashes when taking lomatium alone; however, when it is taken in combination with other herbs which stimulate excretion of waste products, such as dandelion, osha or elder, there are no skin reactions.

Marshmallow   *(Althaea officinalis)*
Part used: Root, leaf and flower
Actions: Demulcent, anti-inflammatory, emollient, expectorant, vulnerary
Indications: Marshmallow candies were originally made by peeling marshmallow roots to reveal the white pulp, cutting them into chunks and boiling them in sugar water, causing them to swell up and become gelatinous. The resulting mucilaginous candy was given to children for tummy aches and coughs—a far cry from our present-day confection! Marshmallow is a soothing, demulcent and mucilaginous herb used for its cooling and moisturizing effects on the body. For irritated mucous membranes and inflamed tissues, marshmallow reigns supreme. It is useful for ulcers, and its nutritive qualities can aid heartburn and other digestive complaints.

It is soothing for kidney and urinary tract ailments. It can help chronic bladder infections in combination with other vulnerary and antimicrobial herbs such as uva ursi and yarrow. Naturopath Jill Stansbury suggests making a cold infusion of marshmallow by soaking 1 tablespoon of dried roots or fresh leaves or flowers in 1 cup of cold water. For recurrent bladder infections, drink 3 to 6 cups of this tea over the course of 24 hours and then slowly decrease the dose as symptoms improve.

Its moisturizing effects ease respiratory complaints and are often included in formulas for bronchitis and dry, hacking coughs. One study showed that marshmallow enhances phagocytosis, indicating its therapeutic use in gastrointestinal and urinary tract infections and in wound healing. Topically, marshmallow is used as a poultice or compress for treating abrasions, inflammations and rashes.

A marshmallow decoction can be made by simmering 1 teaspoon of chopped marshmallow root in 8 ounces of water for 10 to 15 minutes. Strain, and drink up to three cups daily. It is quite mucilaginous. A tincture of marshmallow can be useful as well, but teas are more effective for urinary tract ailments. The mucilage in marshmallow does not extract well in glycerin or in a high percentage of alcohol, so make a low-alcohol extract or tincture.

Milk Thistle   (Silybum marianum)
Part used: Seed
Actions: Hepatoprotective, demulcent, galactogogue, bitter tonic
Indications: This common thistle contains some of the most powerful liver-protective substances known. In Europe, milk thistle extracts are used intravenously to neutralize the deadly toxins of the amanita mushroom *(Amanita phalloides)* and prevent liver damage. Milk thistle is primarily used to treat liver ailments and even to regenerate liver tissue. It is one of the only effective substances known to treat hepatitis A and B. It is used to treat cirrhosis and to repair liver damage caused by envi-

ronmental toxins, alcohol and other drugs. Many clinical and experimental studies have demonstrated milk thistle's hepatoprotective properties.

Milk thistle acts as an antioxidant in preventing free radical damage and has been shown to be many times more potent than vitamin E in its antioxidant effects. It has great benefit in formulas for combating chronic skin ailments through its powerful yet gentle action as a detoxifier. Milk thistle seed is also protective against the harmful effects of radiation treatments and x-rays. It increases the production of breast milk for nursing mothers. As a bitter tonic, milk thistle improves digestion and promotes the flow of bile.

Milk thistle was formerly used as an antidepressant in conjunction with despondency, apathy and forgetfulness. The liver was often treated in patients with depression, as the liver was associated with melancholia. Its tonic effects are gradual, and greater benefits can be seen by using the herb for at least a three-month period. Even taken in large doses, the only side effects seen are mild laxative effects in isolated cases.

Milk thistle seed is usually taken in doses of ¼ teaspoon of tincture three to six times daily or 2 capsules, two to three times daily. The nutty-tasting seed can also be roasted and ground in a spice mill or coffee grinder, and taken in doses of 2 to 3 tablespoons daily, sprinkled on food.

Nettles   *(Urtica dioica)*
Part used: Leaves, seeds and root
Actions: Tonic, astringent, hemostatic, diuretic, galactagogue, expectorant
Indications: Commonly called stinging nettle, the tiny hairs on the underside of the leaf and stem do indeed produce a stinging sensation when brushed, but the many benefits of nettles seem to outweigh the temporary prickly

itch. The stinging hairs of fresh nettles contain formic acid, but when dried or steamed, the plant acids are neutralized and nettle loses its sting.

Nettle is an excellent blood builder, especially in anemia. Nettle is also used to stop bleeding, both internally and externally. An excellent rejuvenative tonic, nettle improves skin conditions, such as eczema and rashes, and as a tea is useful for inflammatory conditions of the bladder and kidneys, including cystitis. Its high mineral content makes it beneficial for overcoming fatigue and raising low energy levels.

Its nourishing and immune-stimulating properties make it useful for arthritis and gout as well as allergies and hay fever. In Europe an effective, albeit painful, treatment for arthritis involves flogging the arthritic area with a bouquet of nettles. Herbal authority, James Duke, Ph.D. claims that this treatment, called *urtication,* helped eliminate the gout pain in his elbow.

Nettle is also given as a expectorant in respiratory conditions, and recent double-blind studies have demonstrated freeze-dried nettle's effectiveness in the treatment and prevention of allergy symptoms.

Young, spring-gathered nettles have long been a traditional tonic, and their chlorophyll content ranks among the highest of all green plants. Nettle is considered a safe plant, especially in teas or infusions. Young spring nettles are considered best, as hard mineral conglomerates concentrated in older nettles can be irritating to the kidneys.

Nettle tea is usually made by infusing 1 to 2 teaspoons of dried leaf in 8 ounces of water. Drink 1 cup, three times daily. The suggested dose for tincture is 1 or 2 teaspoons diluted in water, three times daily. Another delicious way to enjoy nettles is to steam them, as you would spinach, and add to other dishes such as rice and grains, pasta, omelets, casseroles and stews. Fresh nettle juice is excellent for weak and debilitated persons, and nettle seeds are also beneficial.

Osha
(*Ligusticum porteri*)

Part used: Root

Actions: Antiviral, diaphoretic, expectorant, anti-inflammatory, bitter, immunostimulant, diuretic, anti-bacterial

Indications: Osha is a highly aromatic herb in the carrot (*umbelliferae*) family, which grows at high altitudes in the southwestern states. Commonly used for a wide range of ailments, osha is a strong immune stimulant and superb remedy for viral infections, especially taken at the first sign of symptoms. It is a specific for acute bronchial infections and inflammation, sore throat and dry irritated cough with painful expectoration. Its diaphoretic action brings about elimination of toxins through sweating. Its anesthetizing properties soothe pain in the chest due to coughing and expectoration.

Osha root is excellent in cough syrups. Southwest herbalist Michael Moore suggests grinding the root and placing it in a pot. Cover the root with twice as much honey. Heat gently for one hour. Cool slightly, and strain through cheesecloth. Another method is to add 1 ounce of osha tincture to 3 ounces of prepared herbal cough syrup made from mullein, sage and wild cherry bark.

As a bitter, osha aids indigestion and helps recuperation when there has been vomiting; it relieves flatulence and its antibacterial properties help gastrointestinal infections.

This herb is helpful for edema, and its diuretic qualities aid in reducing urine retention. Osha is quite useful in the initial stages of a cold or in treating allergies when there is copious clear mucus. Topically, osha can be used as an antibacterial on superficial infections and can effectively reduce simple inflammation due to bug bites, stings and skin rashes.

Some find the taste of osha harsh and overpowering, but I think it can be best described as a flavor akin to strong, bitter celery. Since osha's constituents are not very readily soluble in water, tinctures or capsules work best. As a recommended dose for an acute stage of the above conditions, take 10 to 15 drops of tincture every hour. For chronic conditions, 30 to 40 drops every three to four hours up to five times a day is helpful. If using capsules, take 1 capsule every three to four hours. Osha is contraindicated in pregnancy, as carrot family plants might cause miscarriage.

Pau D'arco   *(Tabebuia spp.)*
Part used: Inner bark
Actions: Antifungal, antibacterial, antimicrobial, antiviral, antiparasitic, anti-inflammatory
Indications: This South American tree has quite a number of common names, including lapacho, taheebo, ipes, trumpet bush and in Brazil, where it is used medicinally, it is known as ipe roxo. Widely acclaimed as a folk remedy, pau d'arco has significant antibiotic and antifungal properties. A long list of ailments for which it is used by the native Indians of Brazil includes boils, dysentery, ulcers, fever, snakebites, syphilis, wounds, cancer of the esophagus, lung and prostate, arthritis, cystitis and respiratory conditions. And the list goes on. Can pau d'arco really be the miracle plant that folk healers claim it to be? Scientific research, including both animal and human studies is showing us that perhaps it can.

It is clearly successful against *Candida albicans, Staphylococcus, Trichophyton,* malaria and tuberculosis. Its antiviral activity has demonstrated effects against herpes Types 1 and 2, and it is being studied for use against HIV and chronic fatigue syndrome. Pau d'arco's ability to destroy bacteria, viruses, parasites and fungi is apparently due to the fact that it increases oxygen supply at the local level. Most well-known, however, is its antifungal use. Clinical herbalist and author, Dr. Terry Willard, says that he has had great results in treating yeast infections with pau d'arco tea, and in cases of vaginitis, with suppositories or tampons soaked in lapacho tea.

Pau d'arco has also been reputed to be an antitumor remedy ever since a 1968 study, when lapachol was shown to be among the most important antitumor substances derived from plants. More recent research has shown only mild antitumor effects, although lapacho's role as an immune stimulant has been validated.

A tea or decoction is the traditional way of using pau d'arco. An effective dose is 2 to 6 cups of decoction daily, made by pouring 2 to 3 cups of cold water over 1 tablespoon of the herb. Simmer for 10 minutes, strain and drink. Ten to 30 drops of tincture, taken two to eight times daily is the equivalent dose of tincture. There have been no reports of toxicity to humans.

Red Clover *(Trifolium pratense)*
Part used: Flower heads
Actions: Alterative, expectorant, antispasmodic, antitussive, antibiotic
Indications: As children, we used to suck the honey-sweet nectar from the red clover blossoms on a sunny summer day, never realizing that it is one of the best remedies for childhood skin diseases such as eczema and psoriasis. Topically, it is a popular ingredient in salves for skin sores. A mild and delicious tasting herb, red clover has a high mineral content and gentle antitussive and expectorant effects, making it a good choice for infections such as bronchitis and debilitating conditions.

Ex-coal miner Harold Hoxsey used red clover as an ingredient in his famous Hoxsey Formula for cancer from the 1930s to the 1950s, and hundreds of his patients claimed that this formula cured their cancers. The Hoxsey formula is still available today at the Bio-Medical Center in Tijuana, Mexico, and many contemporary herbalists in the United States manufacture similar products.

Red clover is considered safe and nontoxic, but its estrogenic plant sterols have been the source of concern for some who question its use as a treatment in estrogen-dependent cancers. However, medical herbalist Amanda McQuade Crawford says that red clover can be used as part of a holistic treatment for breast tumors and fibroids because its sterols compete with excess estrogen, thus bringing the body into balance.

Much of the red clover available commercially contains mostly leaves and brown flowers which are of poor quality, and therefore results are unreliable. To ensure good quality, buy from reputable wildcrafters. Island Herbs is an excellent source for high-quality red clover blossoms. See Herbal Suppliers in the Appendix.

To make a tea of red clover, use 1 or 2 teaspoons of dried blossoms to 1 cup of water or 2 ounces dried flowers per quart of water to make an infusion. Drink 1 cup, three times daily. A suggested dose of tincture is 1 teaspoon in water, three times daily. For external use, make a compress or use as a wash.

The only ill effects reported from the use of red clover are minor discomforts such as stomach upset or flatulence. This may largely be due to using red clover products containing mostly leaves. Since red clover is in the legume (pea and bean) family, flatulence may result from compounds in the leaf.

Reishi *(Ganoderma spp.)*
Part used: Fruiting body
Actions: Adaptogen, immunostimulant, nervine, antitumor, antiviral, antioxidant, expectorant, anti-inflammatory, antibacterial
Indications: Also known as *ling-zhi* (spirit plant), reishi

has been used in Chinese folk medicine for thousands of years. It is often called the mushroom of immortality and is considered to promote longevity and benefit the heart. Stories about reishi abound, including tales of people traveling long distances to find it and even corpses coming back to life after reishi was placed upon their lips! The cloud-like motifs which adorned the robes of the emperor and even the Great Wall of China are said to be representative of this mushroom.

A number of clinical studies have been done over the past 20 years showing reishi's benefit for many disorders including heart and lung ailments, insomnia, allergies, duodenal ulcers, Alzheimer's disease, diabetes, high blood pressure and high cholesterol. It contributes to pain relief, protects the liver in hepatic disease and is a powerful scavenger of free radicals, thereby slowing the aging process. Its effectiveness seems to be due to the collective action of many of its components including the polysaccharides which have immunostimulating activity.

Reishi has been shown to raise T-cell levels and is used as a superior immune tonic, especially in Asia. It is considered a specific for chronic fatigue syndrome, has been used as a treatment for immune disorders such as AIDS and cancer, and can protect against the effects of radiation. Its adaptogenic qualities make it useful for stress. Its antimicrobial effects inhibit bacteria, fungi and viruses.

One of its more unique features is its ability to treat altitude sickness by oxygenating the blood. Although not clearly understood, research shows that reishi's antiallergic effects stem from compounds which inhibit the release of histamine.

In *Medicinal Mushrooms,* Christopher Hobbs gives the following method for preparing a liquid extract of reishi (or other dried medicinal mushrooms). Reishi's tough, woody consistency lends itself to this method of preparation, and it makes a good tonic for long-term use.

Reishi Mushroom Liquid Extract

Place chopped, dried mushrooms in a blender and cover with 80-proof or 100-proof vodka. Blend until it is the consistency of a fruit smoothie. Pour into a quart or ½-gallon canning jar. After 30 minutes, the mushroom pieces will sink to the bottom and there will be about an inch of clear liquid at the top of the jar. Make sure no pieces of mushroom stick up above the liquid. Shake the bottle each day and keep it in a warm place away from direct light. Strain after two weeks, squeezing as much liquid as possible from the mushroom pulp. (This is a simple tincture.) Pour the liquid tincture back into a clean jar with a lid. Now, place the mushroom pulp in a pot and cover with five times as much water. Simmer for 1 hour. Cool and then strain and squeeze as much liquid from the pulp as possible. Compost the pulp. Pour the liquid decoction back in the pot and simmer until it is reduced to ⅕ of its original volume. Add this concentrate back to the original tincture, making sure that this final preparation contains at least 20 to 25 percent alcohol. (You can calculate this based upon the percentage of alcohol in the first tincture.) Hobbs says that this preparation is "richer in the immune-activating and antitumor polysaccharides, as well as the protein-bound polysaccharides and will be more tonifying than the original alcohol preparation."

An effective dose of reishi is ½ to 2 teaspoons of the above preparation twice daily in water or ginger tea, or 3 tablets, three times a day. Reishi mushroom is considered nontoxic and safe to use. Rare side effects are upset stomach after long-term use.

Schisandra   (Schisandra chinensis)
Part used: Fruit
Actions: Tonic, astringent, sedative, antibacterial, hepatoprotective, antidepressant, antiallergenic, adaptogenic

Indications: The fruit of schisandra is a bright red peppercorn-sized berry which grows in grape-like bunches on a hardy perennial vine. Although rare in American gardens, this valuable fruit is commonly grown in English and Western European gardens. Known as "five-flavor berry," it is considered balanced in the sense that its unique taste comes from berries that are sweet, sour, bitter, salty and pungent.

Schisandra is available as a dried berry in natural food stores in the United States or in Chinese markets, where it is known as *Wu-wei-zi*. Even though this herb is only beginning to gain popularity in the West, it has been used widely in traditional Chinese medicine (TCM) as an astringent tonic and adaptogen with liver-protecting effects similar to milk thistle. Somewhat weaker in its action than *Panax* or Siberian ginseng, it has the ability to help one retain energy, improve mental capacity, increase endurance and build strength.

A strong antioxidant, it is used in TCM for liver conditions such as hepatitis and to counter the ill effects of chemical toxins on the liver, especially carbon tetrachloride. It stimulates glycogen production in the liver, calms the nervous system, and counteracts the stimulating effects of caffeine. As a respiratory tonic, it treats coughs, wheezing, asthma and lung weakness. It has been shown to have blood sugar-regulating effects and alleviate night sweats. Hunting tribes in Northern China and Eastern Siberia eat schisandra berries to provide them with strength and energy on long forays. In Russia, schisandra is a registered medicine for vision problems and astigmatism.

Schisandra is considered a very safe tonic herb which may be helpful in many immune-related conditions. The only contraindications are for those with epilepsy and in severe hypertension. The standard dose for schisandra is 3 to 9 grams in decoction.

Shiitake *(Lentinus edodes)*

Part used: Fruiting body

Actions: Immune regulator, antitumor, antiviral, hypotensive, adaptogen, anti-inflammatory, hepatoprotective, antibacterial, antiparasitic

Indications: Shiitake mushroom has long been used in Asia as both food and medicine. Unlike the tough, woody reishi, shiitake is a tender, succulent and delicious mushroom and can be cooked and eaten in many dishes. "Shiitake" literally means "shii fungus" or mushroom which grows on shii (a species of oak) trees. Until about 1972, only dried shiitake was available in the United States, but it is now cultivated here and is widely available in the produce section of most supermarkets.

Shiitake has both antiviral and immune-enhancing properties that makes it beneficial to people with chronic viral infections, those with cancer and AIDS and those with depressed immunity. Lentinan, a highly valuable, nontoxic compound in shiitake, is a powerful immune-enhancer with antiviral effects that have proved stronger than the prescription drug amantadine hydrochloride in its capability to fight viruses and tumor cells. One reason for this is that it increases interferon activity and stimulates production of antibodies and white blood cells. Studies at Budapest's Institute of Pathology and Experimental Cancer Research showed lentinan's ability to inhibit metastasis to the lung. The study demonstrated that through the use of this shiitake compound, immune cells can be stimulated to increase both their numbers and their activity against tumor cells. In Japan, it is considered so valuable that pure lentinan is given intravenously to patients for immune disorders.

Studies show that both the mushroom and its mycelium (the underground network of thread-like fibers from which it grows) are important for their medicinal effects. Shiitake has been shown to lower blood pressure and cholesterol in human studies, to produce antibodies to hepatitis B and to improve liver function in mice. Human studies also demonstrate its capacity to reduce bronchial inflammation, help urinary incontinence and, according to Christopher Hobbs, LEM (*Lentinula edodes* mycelium extract) may be more effective than AZT in the treatment of AIDS and far less expensive, at a cost of about $74 per month for a therapeutic dose of 3 grams daily. Shiitake is also used effectively for candida infections, frequent colds and flu and environmental allergies.

The traditional therapeutic dose for benefiting immunity is 6 to 16 grams of the dried mushroom or 90 grams of the fresh fruiting body. Standardized extracts are also available and are more beneficial than tablets, since the amount of lentinan is certified and clearly stated. For immune maintenance, eating shiitake regularly is beneficial. No toxicity is known for shiitake, but the mushroom must be cooked, since ingesting the fresh, raw mushroom may cause digestive upsets. An excellent source for fresh, certified organically grown shiitake mushrooms is DelfTree Farm in North Adams, Massachusetts.

St. Johnswort *(Hypericum perforatum)*
Part used: Unopened buds and flowering tops
Actions: Antispasmodic, anti-inflammatory, vulnerary, antiviral, antidepressant, alterative, diuretic, anthelmintic, antibacterial
Indications: For more than 2,000 years, St. Johnswort has been used for wound healing, damaged nerves and as a diuretic and astringent. Only recently have scientists begun to study its immune-stimulating effects and use as an antidepressant and antiviral. In more than 25 clinical trials, it was shown to be an effective antidepressant. Steven Foster reports that in a placebo-controlled double-blind study of 105 patients diagnosed with mild to moderate depression, subjects were given 300 mg of standardized St. Johnswort

extract or a placebo for four weeks. It was found that 67 percent of the treatment group improved, while only 28 percent of the placebo group showed a response. No side effects were seen.

The sedative and pain-relieving effects of this sunny yellow flowering herb are well-substantiated for treatment of anxiety, muscle tension and neuralgia along with sciatica and rheumatic pain. A combination tincture of equal parts St. Johnswort and skullcap (*Scutellaria lateriflora*), taken in ½- to 1-teaspoon doses is quite effective for tension headaches and muscle pain. This dose also helps to alleviate symptoms of anxiety, tension and pain associated with the menstrual cycle and PMS. St. Johnswort is also indicated for menopausal symptoms such as anxiety, mood swings and depression.

Because of its antiviral effects, the herb is being studied for use in HIV/AIDS. Amanda McQuade Crawford reports successful results using a tincture of *Hypericum perforatum* with AIDS patients. The National Cancer Institute has credited St. Johnswort as having potential cancer-fighting effects, with one study showing the ability of mice to fight off the feline leukemia virus with a single dose.

Topically, St. Johnswort works well as an oil or lotion for speeding the healing of strains and sprains as well as bruises, wounds and burns. St. Johnswort oil is also effective for sunburn and seems to be a fairly good sunscreen as well.

There is some question about the safety of St. Johnswort for internal use. If you are fair-skinned, err on the safe side and avoid taking St. Johnswort internally when you will be spending time in bright sun.

The fresh herb seems to produce the best results therapeutically. Extracts standardized to 0.3 percent hypericin are taken in doses of 300 mg three times a day to deliver 1 mg of hypericin daily. Make a tea by using 1 or 2 teaspoons of the dried herb. Pour 8 ounces of boiling water over the herb and steep 15 minutes. Drink three times daily. The tincture can be taken in ¼- to 1-teaspoon doses, three times daily.

One of the unique features of St. Johnswort tincture or oil is its bright burgundy red color produced by the flavonoid hypericin in the plant. If you crush a fresh flower bud between your fingers, this red juice will be released. When making or buying tinctures and oils of St. Johnswort, this rich, red color should be apparent. If the product is pink or pale-colored, the product is inferior.

When making a tincture or oil of St. Johnswort, make sure to first crush the flowers and buds in a blender or food processor or with a mortar and pestle.

Usnea or Old Man's Beard   (*Usnea spp.*)
Part used: Whole lichen
Actions: Antifungal, antispasmodic, antibacterial, antiparasitic, antimicrobial, antibiotic
Indications: Usnea is an excellent antimicrobial herb, and although it is not as easy to find as many of the herbs covered here, it deserves mention. Usnea hangs from trees in gray-green beard-like masses along the coast of Maine and throughout the forests of the Pacific Northwest. It is effective in formulas for fungal conditions such as athlete's foot, yeast infections, respiratory and urinary tract infections. According to herbalist Christopher Hobbs, usnea has been used for stomach weakness, infections of the mucous membranes, dysentery and diarrhea.

Usnea has been shown to have immune-enhancing properties and to improve resistance to colds and flu. In addition, usnic acid, a component of the lichen is effective against staphylococcus and streptococcus, making it useful for some types of skin ailments and sore throats. Hobbs suggests its use in bronchitis, bacterial infection, mastitis, pneumonia, ringworm, sinus infection, urinary tract infection, tuberculosis and the vaginal infection, *trichomonas*.

Usnea is not very water-soluble, and so is best used in a tincture or in an oil base. It is tremendously effective for strep throat and can eliminate the need for antibiotics. As usnea has a rather bitter flavor, the tincture is more palatable when diluted in a small amount of grapefruit juice.

Herbalist Deb Soule gives a simple, but powerful immune-stimulating formula in her book, *The Roots of Healing*. Make a tincture of equal parts lomatium, usnea, echinacea root and goldenseal root. Take 25 to 50 drops, three to five times a day. She suggests using this formula for seven to ten days at a time for bronchitis, pneumonia, flu, candida, skin lesions, and colds, and in conjunction with other therapies for HIV, herpes and chronic fatigue syndrome.

Usnea ointments and salves are commonly used topically in Europe for fungal infections.

Wild Indigo   *(Baptisia tinctora)*

Part used: Root and leaves
Actions: Antimicrobial, lymphatic, antiseptic, laxative, immunostimulant
Indications: Wild indigo is an immune system stimulant especially indicated when infection or abscess is present. It is one of the first herbs to consider in treating swollen lymph glands. It is indicated in mumps, pelvic inflammatory disease, Epstein Barr virus, infectious mononucleosis and pleurisy. It is a specific for tonsillitis and infectious conditions of the upper respiratory tract. It is the herb of choice for chronic or recurring infections, such as cystitis and for smoldering inflammation and swampy conditions that you just can't seem to kick. Whenever there is disintegration or death of tissue, wild indigo is specific.

Murray and Pizzorno write in the *Encyclopedia of Natural Medicine,* that baptisia (wild indigo) ''can enhance white-cell destruction of viruses and bacteria, production and activation of lymph cells and the production of anti-bodies." Since it can be toxic in high doses, it should be used with care. Herbalist Kathi Keville says that wild indigo "stimulates production of lymph cells and then gives them a kick in the pants to get them going." Wild indigo has an acrid and somewhat bitter taste, more tolerable in tincture form than tea. It can also be used as an ointment on infected sores.

Because of its potential toxicity, it is best used in combination with other herbs. The side effects of an overdose are vomiting and diarrhea. The suggested dose for the tincture is 2 to 20 drops in a small amount of water. For a large, robust person, the dose might be 20 to 25 drops, whereas for a fragile person the dose would be 2 to 8 drops. For best results, take it three to five times a day, between meals, diluted in a little water. Follow with a glass of water.

Yucca *(Yucca spp.)*
Part used: Root
Actions: Anti-inflammatory, laxative
Indications: Yucca's medicinal use is primarily as an anti-inflammatory and pain reliever, especially for arthritic conditions. This is not the same potato-like tuber sold in the produce section of many supermarkets, but the root of the common southwest plant with long, narrow spiny-tipped leaves. Yucca is known as Spanish bayonet, Spanish dagger and amole in its native habitat of the southwestern United States, where it is used as a popular folk medicine.

A strong coarse fiber is made from the leaves and stalk of the plant and used in the production of rope, baskets, shoes and even washcloths with a texture similar to a loofa sponge. The outer bark of the root is rich in saponin compounds which create a sudsy detergent, useful in washing clothing and hair.

Several clinical studies have been done with arthritic

patients in which one group was given yucca and the other group, a placebo. The group that had taken the yucca reported three times greater results with reduced swelling and less stiffness and pain, even though it took anywhere from a few days to over three months to realize these effects. Because long-term use of yucca is needed to achieve maximum benefit, most of these studies show little action. Kathi Keville reports that when a two-month study was conducted in France with people who had various types of arthritis, the subjects each took 1-½ grams of yucca daily and nine out of ten reported a decrease in the intensity of their pain. The tea may also be effective for inflammation of the prostate.

Make a tea by simmering ¼ ounce of the inner root in 16 ounces of water for 15 minutes and drink three to four doses over the course of the day. The suggested dose for tablets is 2 tablets taken with meals, three times daily. Yucca is considered a non-toxic herb, but laxative effects can result when drinking copious amounts of the tea.

Common Immune System Ailments

Do you feel drained of energy? Do you collapse in a heap in front of the TV at night, too exhausted to do anything else? A weakened immune system may be why you are too pooped to participate, why that little cut took two weeks to heal, or why every cold or flu going around your neighborhood seems to find you and not want to leave.

The inability to cope with everyday stress, poor nutrition, the chemicals in household cleaners, pesticides in the environment, and antibiotics and hormones in meat and dairy foods may be what's constantly challenging your immune system and getting you down.

The list of ailments linked to a weak immune system seems nearly endless. To do justice to them all would be far beyond the scope of this book. Thus, I have omitted complex immune system challenges such as cancer, AIDS and autoimmune ailments. Resources for more information on these conditions are included in the reference section. Herbal treatments for some of the more common —and less life-threatening—immune system conditions are featured in this chapter.

CANDIDIASIS

The common yeast, *Candida albicans* is present in every person's body—in the gastrointestinal tract, on the skin and, in women, in the vagina. This is a harmless micro-organism when it occurs in normal amounts. It is only when an overgrowth of this yeast occurs that a problem develops.

Some of the common symptoms of candidiasis are chronic fatigue, intestinal cramping, bloating, frequent belching, appetite loss, general malaise, allergies, chronic or recurring vaginal yeast infections, PMS, depression, foggy thinking and irritability. No wonder the diagnosis of candidiasis is often difficult!

Most often, candidiasis is concentrated in the digestive tract, sometimes involving a condition called ''leaky gut.'' This occurs when the intestinal wall becomes too porous, leaking undigested proteins into the blood which, in turn, increases the risk of food allergies. When the immune system is already compromised, as in people with AIDS or in those undergoing chemotherapy, candida can become systemic, traveling to other parts of the body via the blood. This can manifest as thrush (candida overgrowth of the mouth), inability to concentrate and chemical sensitivities as well as other symptoms.

Candida overgrowth is most often associated with chronic use of antibiotics which destroy much of the intestinal flora or ''friendly bacteria'' of the digestive tract, which keep candida in balance. What makes candidiasis such a tough nut to crack is that it is usually not diagnosed until it becomes systemic. *Important:* Women with recurring or chronic yeast infections should be tested for HIV before they decide to self-medicate. Chronic yeast infections are one of the most common presenting complaints in women with HIV.

Although the problem of candida overgrowth (candidiasis) has been around for a very long time, it has only been since William Crook published *The Yeast Connection* in 1984 that the magnitude of this ailment has become apparent. Many people with chronic candidiasis have a wide range of different symptoms, depending on predisposing factors, including age, sex, diet, drug use and impaired immunity.

According to Murray and Pizzorno, the typical candidiasis patient is an adult female between the ages of 15 and 50. She has a history of chronic vaginal yeast infections and has used antibiotics to treat either infections or acne. She uses birth control pills or perhaps an oral steroid hormone. She may have PMS as well as food and chemical sensitivities along with other allergies. She craves carbohydrates or other foods rich in yeast and could have psoriasis, irritable bowel syndrome or other hormonally related problems.

A multidimensional approach is important in treating candidiasis. The first step is to eliminate the use of antibiotics, steroids, birth control pills and drugs which are immune suppressants. Next, enhance digestion with digestive supplements taken with meals such as hydrochloric acid (HCL) capsules, pancreatin, 250 to 500 mg of bromelain or 500 to 1,000 mg of papain. Acidophilus capsules may help to restore the friendly bacteria in the gut, and some find yogurt (made with acidophilus culture) helpful as well. Swedish bitters can be another helpful digestive aid.

Support liver function (and digestion with 1 to 1-½ teaspoons dandelion tincture, taken three times daily, or dandelion capsules, 4 grams, three times daily. Another way to help the liver is to sprinkle 1 tablespoon of ground milk thistle seed (*Silybum marianum*) on food at each meal. The seed may be ground in a coffee grinder or spice mill with any extra stored in the freezer.

Another essential step is a diet to control candidiasis. It is of utmost importance to eliminate all sugars including honey, maple syrup and fruit juices since candida yeast thrives on sugars. Other dietary recommendations are to avoid foods with a high yeast or mold content such as yeasted breads, cheese, dried fruits, melons, peanuts and all alcoholic beverages, since they promote yeast overgrowth. All milk products should be avoided as well because of their high milk sugar (lactose) and antibiotic content. Eliminate foods which cause digestive upsets, since they are likely to be allergens which weaken the immune system and provide a place for yeast to thrive. Also, limit foods high in carbohydrates, like potatoes and corn. Some people find that they cannot tolerate leftovers, since any foods over a day old can encourage candida growth. These individuals should cook what they plan to eat that day and freeze leftovers immediately.

So, what can be eaten? All vegetables are fine (with the exception of those already mentioned above), protein sources (it's best to buy organic or naturally raised meats), and whole grains as well as two or three 1-cup servings daily of fresh apples, berries, pears or cherries.

Finally, support the immune system with herbs and nutritional supplements which control yeast overgrowth and help friendly intestinal flora to flourish. Antifungal herbs are most important. Garlic tops the list, being more effective against *C. albicans* than Nystatin and most other antifungal drugs. Besides using it liberally in foods, garlic capsules should be taken daily. Kwai or other unheated garlic works best. Echinacea has been used to successfully inhibit candida and yeast infection. In one study, maximum results were achieved when echinacea extract was taken for 10 weeks.

Both pau d'arco and black walnut show strong anti-fungal activity for candidiasis, and they support the immune system as well. Barberry and Oregon grape have immune-stimulating capabilities. Both contain berberine, a valuable compound which fights a wide range of micro-organisms including *Candida albicans*. Many common, aromatic spices also have powerful antifungal properties. These include cloves, allspice, cinnamon, ginger, thyme and rosemary. These can be used creatively in cooking, and teas of lemon balm, lavender or chamomile are also helpful.

Here is an excellent anti-candida tincture from herbalist Kathi Keville.

Candida Tincture

1 ounce tincture of black walnut husk (must be fresh)
½ ounce each tinctures of lavender flowers, valerian root and pau d'arco
10 drops tea tree essential oil

Combine ingredients and shake well before using. Take 2 to 3 droppersful a day.

Or, try my formula:

Last, But Not Yeast Tincture

2 parts each tinctures of echinacea, black walnut and pau d'arco
3 parts usnea tincture
1 part each tinctures of barberry *or* Oregon grape root
1 part ginger

Combine all tinctures together. Then add 2 drops of garlic flower essence and 2 drops of chaparral flower essence to each ounce of tincture. Take ¼ to ½ teaspoon in water three times daily.

CHRONIC FATIGUE AND IMMUNE DYSFUNCTION SYNDROME (CFIDS)

Once called "yuppie flu" because of its common occurrence among young, hard-working, upwardly mobile individuals (primarily women) and because sufferers have flu-like symptoms, this complex condition of the immune system is not well understood. Chronic Epstein Barr Virus (EBV) Syndrome, and myalgic encephalomyelitis (ME) are some of the other names for this puzzling condition whose broad symptom picture includes fatigue, recurrent sore throats, low-grade fever, insomnia, lymph node swelling, muscle and joint pain, headache, memory loss, depression, anxiety, blurry vision, multiple allergies, rashes, intestinal discomfort, impaired concentration, recurrent respiratory infections and sometimes additional complaints as well. Ninety five percent have fatigue as their primary symptom, and ninety percent have cognitive function disorders; that is, they have fuzzy thinking and difficulty translating thoughts into words.

The cause is not known, and diagnosis can be extremely difficult since other disorders such as parasitic and autoimmune diseases, Lyme disease, lymph diseases and heavy-metal poisoning can have similar symptoms. To make matters even more complicated, many other diseases—especially allergies and *Candida albicans*—coexist with CFIDS. It is also thought that *Giardia lamblia,* and *Trichomonas* may be associated with CFIDS. We do know that stress and weakened immunity are key predisposing factors. The overuse of anti-hypertensives, tranquilizers and anesthetics may be other cofactors.

Fibromyalgia, another ailment with very similar symptoms but with more muscle involvement and pain, may actually be another form of CFIDS. Although not an anti-inflammatory disease per se, fibromyalgia is a condition of muscle tenderness and stiffness with "trigger points" of more acute inflammation and pain. It is more common in women than in men and occurs more in young women who are stressed, anxious, depressed, tense and striving. Those diagnosed with fibromyalgia usually feel better after exercise, while those with CFIDS usually feel worse with exercise.

Experts agree that EBV is a member of the herpes group

of viruses, including *herpes simplex* 1 and 2, cytomegalo-virus and *Varicella zoster*. After the initial infection, these viruses can remain dormant for a lifetime, kept in check by a healthy immune system. When the immune system is weakened or compromised, however, these viruses can become reactivated, causing the symptoms listed above. Because impaired adrenal function is common among those with CFIDS, it is now suspected that CFIDS may start with adrenal exhaustion. An alarming fact is that CFIDS is on the rise, and this syndrome can persist from months to many years.

So, how do we begin to treat this enigma? The first and most vital step is to enhance immune system function. Start by eliminating allergens and chemicals in the diet and/or environment. This includes drugs, heavy metals, overgrowth of *Candida albicans,* food allergens and other pathogens which tax the immune system and eliminative organs. Next, stimulate blood flow to the lymphatic system with massage, exercise and lymphatic herbs. Support the immune system with a diet consisting of organically grown whole foods which are low in fat and high in fiber, moderate amounts of high quality protein and complex carbohydrates. Include lightly steamed vegetables, fresh, ripe fruits and eight to ten glasses of pure water daily. Nutrient-dense foods such as spirulina, garlic, seaweeds, burdock, nettles and oats are beneficial, as well as a good bioavailable multi-vitamin mineral supplement and the enzyme Co-Q 10. Vitamin C plays an important role, with its antiviral activity and ability to increase resistance to infection. If *C. albicans* is involved, a candida diet as described on pages 67-68 of this book is a must. Of course, exercise (within the capacity of the individual) and stress management techniques are vital.

Some herbs to consider in the treatment of CFIDS include immunomodulators such as echinacea, Oregon grape root, barberry or goldenseal, adrenal tonics like Siberian ginseng, astragalus, cleavers or licorice, unless high blood pressure or edema is present.

Lomatium and red root are also indicated for lymph congestion, swollen glands and viral conditions. Milk thistle and schisandra both support liver function. Bitter digestive tonics are helpful, including burdock, and dandelion. Adaptogens like reishi and shiitake are also important. Many other herbs can be used in the treatment of CFIDS, but since symptoms vary somewhat for each person, the most effective formula is one that is geared to each individual's unique symptoms.

The following formula may be helpful in treating fibromyalgia and CFIDS.

Fibromyalgia Tincture
2 parts echinacea (*Echinacea spp.*)
2 parts yucca root (*Yucca spp.*)
2 parts black cohosh (*Cimicifuga racemosa*)
1 part devil's claw (*Harpagophytum procumbens*)
1 part cleavers (*Galium aparine*)
1 part dandelion (*Taraxacum officinale*)
1 part licorice root (*Glycyrrhiza glabra*)

Combine tinctures. Take 1 teaspoon in water three times a day.

For pain and inability to sleep, the formula below may prove beneficial.

Pain and Insomnia Tincture
3-½ parts valerian (*Valeriana officinalis*)
3-½ parts Jamaican dogwood (*Piscidia erythrina*)
1 part St. Johnswort (*Hypericum perforatum*)
1 part skullcap (*Scutellaria laterifolia*)
1 part chamomile (*Matricaria recutita*)

Combine tinctures. Take ½ teaspoon in water as needed.

Flower Essence Formula for CFIDS

Self-Heal (for confidence and trust in one's own ability to get well)

Lavender (for nervous tension leading to depletion and exhaustion)

Olive (for deep exhaustion on all levels)

Aloe vera (for burn-out from overuse or misuse of creative forces)

To make a dosage bottle, combine 2 drops of each stock flower essence in a 1 ounce dropper bottle of spring water. Take 4 drops as needed.

COLDS AND FLU

We are forever seeking the cure for the common cold, and faster than we can keep up with the latest strain of flu, a new, more highly evolved one seems to be lurking just around the corner. So what can be done to stay well and protect against the next cold or flu that's going around?

First and foremost, it is important to maintain a healthy immune system by eating well, reducing stress and avoiding junk foods, chemical additives, pollutants, drugs, cigarettes and other substances known to suppress immunity. Both colds and flu involve respiratory symptoms such as sore throats, coughs, sneezing, congested sinuses, headache, muscle aches and fatigue. But the flu is usually more severe and can involve fever, vomiting and/or diarrhea. For most healthy adults, colds and flu are bothersome and inconvenient, but symptoms usually last for about a week or so and then improve on their own. However, for very young children, the elderly and those whose immune systems are already compromised, these ailments can be life-threatening. With a little herbal help, recovery may occur in much less time than generally thought possible. Or, better yet, one can stop a cold or flu from coming on by treating the earliest symptoms.

There's good reasoning behind the usual advice to "drink fluids and get plenty of rest." The immune system functions better when one is asleep. Potent immune-enhancing compounds are released by the body during the deepest levels of sleep. With a cold, the mucous membranes of the respiratory tract get dehydrated. This provides a hospitable environment in which the virus thrives. By drinking fluids (particularly herbal teas, water and dilute fruit juices), the respiratory tract is moisturized and the virus is repelled. Drinking orange juice (which is high in fruit sugar) does more harm than good, since sugar impairs white blood cell function and inhibits immunity. It is best to drink juice diluted with water; grapefruit and lemon juice are especially good, as are vegetable juices and soups.

Taking 500 to 1,000 mg of vitamin C with bioflavonoids every couple of hours is very helpful. If diarrhea develops, cut back on the dose. An effective dose of vitamin A is 25,000 units each day. One 23-mg zinc lozenge every two waking hours for up to one week is beneficial as well.

Echinacea is #1, garlic is #2, and goldenseal is #3 on the list of the 10 most popular herbs in the United States today. All three of these herbs are most often used in this country for colds and flu. While both echinacea and garlic are effective for these conditions, goldenseal is probably wasted in acute infections. When cold or flu symptoms begin, taking up to 1 teaspoon of echinacea tincture every two to three hours can nip it in the bud. Once a cold or flu is well-established, echinacea works better in combination with other herbs, such as boneset, elderberry, or astragalus.

If one is susceptible to colds and flu it is helpful to take echinacea, garlic, astragalus, reishi or shiitake during cold season and during flu season, echinacea, garlic, osha, elderberry juice or boneset. Its best to take small doses after exposure to the flu or a cold and larger doses at the first symptoms of cold or flu.

Boneset (*Eupatorium perfoliatum*) is quite a bitter-tasting herb, which could account for its falling out of popularity in modern herbalism, but it is an important herb to know about. It was once considered the premier remedy for the flu. Because of the aches and pains associated with the flu, it was called "breakbone fever." Boneset was named for its ability to treat this condition. Boneset is best used dried, in a cold infusion for chronic conditions, and as a hot infusion for acute conditions. Because it is such a potent herb, it is best to drink only 1 to 3 ounces of the infusion, rather than a cup. Dr. Fritz Weiss recommends a combination of echinacea and boneset for acute viral infections.

Elderberry flowers (*Sambucus canadensis*) have been used traditionally as a tea for colds, fevers and sore throats. More recently, research has shown that the juice of the berries of black elder (*Sambucus nigra*) not only stimulates the immune system but is effective against eight different influenza viruses. Research from Israel shows that elderberry juice works by preventing flu viruses from replicating. Since the beneficial constituents of black elder are not soluble in alcohol, it is best to drink teas or juice, rather than using a tincture. A syrup made from the juice is available in natural food stores as *Sambucol*. An effective dose of the liquid fruit extract is 40 drops every four hours. It is also available in capsules. No adverse reactions have been seen with elderberry fruit extracts.

Chicken soup has been popular as a remedy for those convalescing from colds and flu in many traditions. Spicy chicken soup is best, especially when made with garlic, onions, chili peppers or curry. A slice or two of astragalus root may be added while the soup is cooking along with some shiitake or maitake mushrooms and burdock root slices. Not only will the soup speed recovery but it will taste delicious, too. Miso as a base for this soup is recommended for vegetarians.

The following recipes (in addition to *Shot-Gun Smoothie,* page 7) are some of my favorites for relieving colds and flu.

Thanks to Rosemary Gladstar, for the following recipe. It is deeply invigorating and clearing to the sinuses. Use it on salads or take a teaspoon every half hour or as needed.

Fire Cider

¼ cup fresh, grated horseradish
⅛ cup garlic, chopped
½ cup onion, chopped
¼ cup fresh, grated ginger
Cayenne and honey to taste
Enough apple cider vinegar to cover all ingredients by 1 to 2 inches

Grate and chop ingredients. Put everything in a glass jar and cover with vinegar. Steep for four weeks. Strain. Sweeten to taste with honey.

Another delicious and effective remedy is *Hot Ginger Lemonade.* See page 7 for the recipe.

When I was 12 years old, I had a severe case of whooping cough. Since my father was a good friend and chiropractic colleague of Dr. George Goodheart, we went to see him for advice. He suggested that I gargle with the following formula, and it worked better to heal my painful, sore throat than anything else I tried.

Dr. George Goodheart's Famous Gargle

1 cup sage tea
2 tablespoons apple cider vinegar

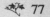

1-2 teaspoons sea salt

Mix all ingredients together. Gargle with the warm tea every half hour for painful sore throats or strep throat. It tastes awful, but the results are worth it.

HERPES SIMPLEX

There are over 100 types of herpes viruses in the herpes family including shingles (*Varicella zoster*), Epstein-Barr (EBV) and cytomegalovirus (CMV). Herpes simplex I is often referred to as "cold sores," with the initial infection commonly occurring in childhood, and recurrent infections appearing throughout adulthood. This infection can remain latent in the body for a lifetime, lying dormant in the nerve ganglia until the immune system is challenged by another infection such as a cold, or by stress, sunburn, pregnancy or menstruation. A poor diet, B-vitamin deficiency, inadequate sleep and use of birth control pills or antibiotics can increase the likelihood of a flare-up. Usually, recurrent infections are less severe than the primary infection.

Outbreaks of oral *Herpes simplex* I generally last two to twelve days, and active shedding of the virus and contagion are possible for the first three to five days. The individual may experience tingling or burning in the area before any lesion is seen.

Herpes simplex II, or genital herpes, usually begins with an itching sensation in the genital area which can last several hours or days before the lesions appear. Reactivation of the infection stimulates the virus to travel the pathway of sensory nerves to the skin, causing blister-like lesions. Blisters erupt within a few days. About 50 percent of those afflicted experience tingling, burning or painful sensations in the genital area as well as back pain. Painful and frequent urination, swelling of the lymph nodes in the groin, headache, fever and systemic illness may also accompany the outbreak. Some people are contagious even when they are asymptomatic.

Although Type I usually occurs "above the belt" and Type II occurs in the genital area, Type I can occasionally cause genital infections, and Type II can cause oral infections. Eventually, outbreaks seem to occur less frequently and may stop after a few years. Dr. Christiane Northrup notes that when an intimate relationship is going well, the immune system seems to function to keep herpes in remission.

The allopathic treatment for herpes is Acyclovir (Zovirax), but there is concern that use of this antiviral medication may result in resistant viral strains that may be harder to treat than the original one. A more holistic approach to this ailment includes immune-strengthening herbs, stress reduction, appropriate diet, exercise and adequate rest.

As far as diet is concerned, foods which are high in arginine should be avoided as they stimulate herpes outbreaks. These include chocolate, peanuts, cashews, almonds, pecans, sesame and sunflower seeds, Brazil nuts, hazelnuts, coconut, walnuts, flaxseeds, buckwheat, peas, corn and cola. Fried, sugary and processed foods should also be eliminated. Emphasize those foods which are high in lysine, such as garlic, brewer's yeast, potatoes and fish. Green leafy vegetables and whole grains are beneficial as well. Focus on an immune-enhancing diet, as discussed on pages 4-8.

Dr. Christiane Northrup suggests that when the familiar "tingling" sensation starts signaling that an outbreak is about to occur, "take 12 capsules of deodorized garlic (available in health food stores) immediately to prevent an outbreak. Then take 3 capsules every four hours while you are awake for the next three days.'' She says that in nearly every case, the herpes outbreak will be prevented. Three cloves of garlic taken twice a day, blended into carrot or vegetable juice, or any other way found palatable, is also helpful.

Beneficial supplements include: 2 grams lysine, 2 to 3 grams vitamin C, 1 gram bioflavonoids, 400 I.U. vitamin E, 15 mg zinc and 50,000 IU beta-carotene, twice daily.

There are many herbs that can bring relief to this painful condition. Echinacea is helpful in 1 teaspoon doses, taken every two hours, as soon as tingling sensations begin. This may prevent an outbreak. Once a herpes outbreak has occurred, 1 dropperful of osha tincture can be taken every three hours. Licorice also has antiviral properties which inhibit the growth and damaging effects of herpes simplex. It can be used internally, as well as topically in a glycyrrhizinic acid ointment, applied three times per day.

St. Johnswort has potent antiviral properties, and is effective both internally and topically for Type I and Type II herpes simplex. In a German study, lemon balm (*Melissa officinalis*) cream applied topically in the very early stages of the herpes infection was very effective in alleviating symptoms and reducing cell damage. Some people find that simply applying ice to the lesions during the early stages of the infection is effective as well. Apply ice for 10 minutes, then take a break for five minutes. Repeat as needed. Topical lysine creams, available in a natural foods store, also provide relief.

To prevent lesions, apply tea tree essential oil to the tingling area with a Q-tip. To dry up lesions, try blending tinctures of calendula, lemon balm, licorice root, echinacea and St. Johnswort, and apply with a Q-tip. Or, blend these tinctures and place in a spray bottle. Add a few drops of essential oils of tea tree and lemon balm. Add enough distilled water to dilute so that it won't sting when you spray it on. This works well for herpes zoster (shingles) as well, which can be extremely painful. Spraying this solution onto the sores is the easiest method of application.

Deb Soule recommends drinking 2 to 4 cups of the following tea daily during a herpes outbreak or whenever a stressful situation occurs:

Nervous System Tea

2 parts oatstraw (*Avena sativa*)
2 parts linden (*Tilia spp.*)
2 parts lemon balm (*Melissa officinalis*)
1 part calendula (*Calendula officinalis*)
1 part nettles (*Urtica dioica*)
1 part skullcap (*Scutellaria lateriflora*)

Place 6 tablespoons of herbs into a glass quart jar and pour boiling water over them. Secure the lid and steep 10 to 20 minutes. Drink throughout the day.

An antiviral tincture can help alleviate symptoms, and if taken early, can prevent an outbreak.

Antiviral Tincture

2 parts St. John's wort (*Hypericum perforatum*)
2 parts echinacea (*Echinacea spp.*)
2 parts calendula (*Calendula officinalis*)
2 parts lemon balm (*Melissa officinalis*)
1 part Siberian ginseng (*Eleutherococcus senticosus*)
1 part licorice (*Glycyrrhiza glabra*)
Self heal flower essence
Garlic flower essence

Combine tinctures. To each ounce of tincture, add 2 drops of each flower essence. Take 1 or 2 droppersful in water, three to four times daily.

URINARY TRACT INFECTIONS

If you have ever had a bout of cystitis or a urinary tract infection (UTI), you will not easily forget it. Typical symptoms are burning, scalding or cloudy urine; increased frequency of urination with a scanty flow; pain with urination; dribbling; straining and urgency. Blood is sometimes present in the urine, but may not be visible and sometimes can only be detected through urinalysis. Cystitis or UTI's are more common in women than in men, and in pregnancy and in post-menopausal women, because the lining of the urethra is thinner. Cystitis is an inflammation and infection of the lining and wall of the bladder. Sometimes called a "bladder infection," this is the most common UTI for women.

Other contributing factors that can make one more susceptible to urinary tract infections are stress, weak immunity, use of antibiotics, resisting the urge to urinate, lack of rest, an enlarged prostate (in men), wearing nylon underwear or tight pants and recent sexual activity with a new partner. Diabetics have high blood sugar, making them more prone to urinary tract infections because the microorganism that causes this ailment thrives on sugar. It is possible for a diabetic's blood sugar to soar out of control if he or she has a urinary tract infection. People who have diabetes and develop a urinary tract infection should seek proper medical care. Hormonal changes caused by oral contraceptives can also initiate infection in some people, and douches, feminine deodorants, sprays and contraceptive jellies and creams can be contributing factors.

Acute cystitis involves inflammation of the lining of the bladder, usually caused by either an infection or obstruction. Accurate diagnosis by a physician is required because if the infection travels up to the kidneys, medical treatment is required. Fever, blood in the urine and/or kidney tenderness are warning signs that the infection may have ascended to the kidneys. If the infection is located in the bladder, herbs and natural therapies can help.

The most common bacteria to cause cystitis is *E. coli*. This bacteria is normally found in the gut, but poor hygiene after a bowel movement or urinating can cause it to travel into the urethral opening. Get into the habit of wiping yourself from front to back after using the toilet. Sexual activity can also irritate the urethra and put pressure on the bladder. Use of a poorly fitting diaphragm or tampon can also be a contributing factor. Those prone to urinary tract infections should be sure to urinate before and after sexual activity.

An appropriate diet is indispensable. It should be light and include dark green leafy vegetables, brown rice and whole grains. If fresh nettles are available, so much the better. Besides their high vitamin and mineral content, blood-building capabilities and overall tonic qualities, nettles are nourishing, strengthening and anti-inflammatory to the kidneys. To cook, steam for 5 minutes (the stinging hairs will instantly dissolve), and serve with brown rice and toasted, ground sesame seeds. Add a dash of tamari or some sea vegetables (like kelp flakes) and garlic, if desired. Other beneficial foods are steamed asparagus, cooked zucchini and yellow squash and watermelon. A low protein diet is necessary, as too much protein is stressful to the kidneys. Cold foods and beverages should be avoided along with coffee, chocolate, black tea and alcohol, as they are all bladder irritants.

Dr. Tori Hudson, Dean of the National College of Naturopathic Medicine says that most people (with the exception of diabetics) get well faster if they fast for a day or two. She also recommends drinking lots of water and unsweetened cranberry juice. Two to four quarts of water a day is about right. Cranberry juice helps to acidify the urine and makes the lining of the bladder "slippery" so that the bacteria can't adhere. Contrary to popular belief, citrus juices are alkalinizing, not acidic, so don't drink citrus juices. Furthermore, the high sugar content of citrus and other sweet juices creates a hospitable environment for the invading microorganisms. Since sweetened cranberry juice creates some of the same problems as other sweet juices, add just enough plain apple juice to the unsweetened cranberry juice to make it palatable. Concentrated cranberry products in capsule form, such as "Cranactin" and other brands, are also effective.

Supplement the diet with 500 mg of vitamin C every hour until acute symptoms subside. Thereafter, 1,000 to 2,000 mg two to three times a day are sufficient. Some people find acidophilus supplements to be helpful, along with 15 mg of zinc daily and 50,000 IU of beta carotene. Many herbs are effective in the treatment of urinary tract infections, but it is necessary to find the right combination for an individual's unique symptoms.

Teas which incorporate herbal diuretics to increase urine production, demulcents to soothe inflamed tissue, astringents to check bleeding, antispasmodics for pain and antimicrobials to stimulate the local immune response in the mucous membranes are also helpful. While tinctures and capsules are easy to take, they are generally less effective than teas in treating UTIs. It is important to drink teas to help to flush out bacteria and microorganisms from the bladder. The following tea is an effective treatment for cystitis and urinary tract infections.

UTI Tea

2 parts nettles (*Urtica dioica*)
2 parts cornsilk (*Zea mays*)
2 parts bearberry (*Arctostaphylos uva-ursi*)
2 parts cleavers (*Galium aparine*)
1 part pipsissewa (*Chimaphila umbellata*)
1 part dandelion greens (*Taraxacum officinalis*)

Combine all dried herbs. Place 1 to 2 teaspoons of this combination in a cup and fill with hot water. Steep 10 to 15 minutes. Drink 1 cup three times daily.

Dr. Tori Hudson's UTI Tincture
Pipsissewa (*Chimaphila umbellata*)
Buchu (*Barosma betulina*)
Bearberry (*Arctostaphylos uva-ursi*)
Horsetail (*Equisetum arvense*)

Combine ¼ ounce of each tincture. Take 20 drops every two hours for two days. If symptoms include lots of burning sensations, combine homeopathic liquid dilutions of apis and cantharis, and take 20 drops of this combination in addition to the formula above. An alternate recommendation for symptoms of burning on urination is to crush 2 homeopathic tablets of cantharis 30x between two pieces of paper. Mix this powder into 8 ounces of water. Take 1 teaspoon per dose, until symptoms improve. Homeopathic remedies are available in natural foods stores.

Some of the most helpful remedies for UTIs are the simplest: drink a quart a day of an infusion of equal parts of cornsilk and nettles; take 2 droppersfuls of echinacea tincture six times a day; take megadoses of vitamin C; drink cranberry juice or take cranberry capsules; and eat steamed nettle greens. Take warm sitz baths and get plenty of rest. Beginning this treatment at the first sign of a urinary tract infection is essential for a quick recovery.

Appendix:

Recommended Reading

Bergner, Paul. *The Healing Power of Echinacea and Goldenseal*. Rocklin, Calif.: Prima Publishing, 1997.

Crook, W. G., *The Yeast Connection*, 2nd Ed., Professional Books, Jackson, Tenn. 1984.

Fulder, Stephen. *How to Survive Medical Treatment*. Essex, England: C. W. Daniel Company Limited, 1994.

Hobbs, Christopher. *Medicinal Mushrooms*. Santa Cruz, Calif.: Botanica Press, 1995.

Hoffmann, David. *Herbs to Relieve Stress*. New Canaan, Conn.: Keats Publishing, Inc., 1996.

———. *The Holistic Herbal*. Dorset, England: Element Books, 1993.

Kaminski, Patricia and Richard Katz. *Flower Essence Repertory*. Nevada City, Calif.: Earth-Spirit, Inc., 1994.

Keville, Kathi. *Herbs for Health Healing*. Emmaus, Pa.: Rodale Press, Inc., 1996.

McQuade Crawford, Amanda. *The Herbal Menopause Book*. Freedom, Calif.: The Crossing Press, 1996.

Moore, Michael. *Medicinal Plants of the Desert and Canyon West*. Santa Fe, N.M.: Museum of New Mexico Press, 1989.

———. *Medicinal Plants of the Mountain West*. Santa Fe, N.M.: Museum of New Mexico Press, 1979.

———. *Medicinal Plants of the Pacific West*. Santa Fe, N.M.: Red Crane Books, 1993.

Moss, Ralph W., Ph.D., *Cancer Therapy: The Independent Consumer's Guide to Non-Toxic Treatment and Prevention*. New York, N.Y.: Equinox Press, 1992.

Murray, Michael, and Joseph Pizzorno. *Encyclopedia of Natural Medicine.* Rocklin, Calif.: Prima Publishing, 1991.

Myss, Caroline, Ph.D., *Anatomy of the Spirit.* New York, N.Y.: Harmony Books, 1996.

Puotinen, CJ. *Herbs for Arthritis.* New Canaan, Conn.: Keats Publishing, Inc., 1997.

Shealy, C. Norman, MD., Ph.D., and Caroline M. Myss, Ph.D., *AIDS: Passageway to Transformation.* Walpole, N.H.: Stillpoint Publishing, 1987.

Soule, Deb. *The Roots of Healing.* New York, N.Y.: Citadel Press, 1995.

Weed, Susun. *Breast Cancer? Breast Health!* Woodstock, N.Y.: Ash Tree Publishing, 1996.

Weil, Andrew, M.D., *Spontaneous Healing.* New York, N.Y.: Alfred A. Knopf, Inc., 1995.

Herbal Suppliers

Avena Botanicals, 219 Mill Street, Rockport, ME 04865.

Delftree Farm, 234 Union Street, North Adams, MA 01247. Growers of fresh, organic shiitake mushrooms.

Eclectic Institute, Inc., 14385 S.E. Lusted Road, Sandy, OR 97055.

Flower Essence Services, P.O. Box 1769, Nevada City, CA 95959.

Frontier Cooperative Herbs, P.O. Box 299, Norway, IA 52318.

Healing Spirits, 9198 St. Rt. 415, Avoca, NY 14809.

Herbalist and Alchemist, P.O. Box 553, Broadway, NJ 08808.

HerbPharm, P.O. Box 116, Williams, OR 97544.

Island Herbs, P.O. Box 25, Waldron Island, WA 98297-0025.

Jean's Greens, 119 Sulpher Springs Road, Newport, NY 13416.

Herbal Directory

The Herbal Green Pages, P.O. Box 245, Silver Spring, MD 17575. One of the most complete resources for products, publications, education, gardens, etc.

INDEX